Die Smiling

Julie Casson

'Julie Casson lays bare the devastating human impact of the UK's ban on assisted dying, capturing precisely why true choice at the end of life is a movement whose time has come for this country. By turns uplifting and heart-wrenching, Die Smiling is a searingly honest tale of love, life and death, and a powerful contribution to a historic debate.'
Sarah Wootton, CEO, Dignity in Dying

Die Smiling

A Memoir: The Sorrows and Joys of a Journey to Dignitas

Julie Casson

Haythorp Books

First published by Haythorp Books, a divison of Canbury Press 2024

This edition published 2024

Haythorp Books

Kingston upon Thames, Surrey, United Kingdom

haythorp.co.uk

Printed and bound in Great Britain

Typeset in Athelas (body), Futura PT (heading)

This is a work of non-fiction

ISBN:

Paperback 9781914487262

Ebook 9781914487255

CONTENTS

Contents

To my family:

Nigel, who will remain forever in my heart.

Craig, Ellie and Becky, who shared the pains, pleasures, perils and triumphs on this journey – a journey nobody should have to make.

And Bodger, who lay patiently by my side as I wrote it all down.

The names of individuals in the caring and medical professions have been changed to respect their privacy.

1
LOOKING BACK

I should never have looked back. Death is ugly. Chilling. It steals the familiar and leaves behind the alien. That beloved face, joyful in life, droops like the muse of tragedy. I didn't realise his lips would turn blue so soon or his skin become waxy and tinged with a purplish hue.

It's not him, my head tells me. He's gone. It's just a corpse. Death has claimed his soul, the living spark of the man I love. Only the vessel for life remains. But my heart wants them to wrap him in a blanket. Please cover him. Keep him warm.

The door to the blue house closes. It's over. What happens now is not my concern. And yet, it is. I stare at the door. Behind it, the escorts will restore the room to its original state. They'll wash the cups and glasses. Place the untouched chocolates back in the box. Secure the lethal gadget in the cupboard from which it came. Safely store the spent syringes, for evidence, until permitted to discard them. One of them, the leader, will notify the police. He'll smoke a couple of fags on the bench outside as he awaits their arrival. An official investigation will follow. The paperwork, so diligently signed, will be complete and in order. Job done. Finished. Exactly what he wanted. Nothing matters now, Julie, does it?

Yes, it matters.

Will they look after him? Will they be gentle? Respectful? Take care not to snag his gastric tube and catheter? How will they lift him from his wheelchair? With no hoist, it will take the strength of two men. What of his coffin? I bet it will be one of those cheap, cardboard, eco things. And then what? How long before he's cremated? Alone. With not a single mourner. Nobody who loves, or cares for him, to guide him on his way. Nobody to place their hand upon his coffin and bow their head in sorrow. Nobody to shed a tear for his loss, and no kind words to mark the life of this brave, funny, exceptional man. The only man I have ever loved. My darling Nigel. My husband.

Nigel believed that without choice, you have nothing.

'I'm lucky,' he said. 'I get to choose how and when I die.'

We will all die. In that, we have no choice. Wouldn't we, if we could, make a deal with Death, and select the option: 'Slip peacefully away in my sleep, right after my hundredth birthday party?' But Death is rarely so generous as to spare us for a century or more, and most pray, when our time comes, it will be swift, and not messy.

When people die, the living search for the mercy in their passing. 'They won't have known anything about it,' we say, when scores perish in a natural disaster. If a mountaineer plunges to his death, 'He died doing what he loved to do.' Following a distressing and painful illness, we are consoled because, 'Their suffering is over.'

There are those who are destined, for a time, to inhabit the world between life and death. Lost in the depths of coma. Neither alive, nor dead. The thing is, they don't know anything about it. That's the merciful part.

Death toyed with Nigel for ten years. Accustomed to its presence, he had no fear of it. In fact, he welcomed it. But Death lingered. Grew bored. As the life dripped from Nigel like water from a tap, Death, perhaps lured by the thrill of devastating catastrophes, dragged its feet.

Nigel was confronted by the rest of his life. His fate was to languish in a world where there is no mercy. Where his astute, tortured mind, entombed in a silenced, paralysed body, would long for Death to remember him. This is a place where, he knew, he would be both alive, and dead.

As I look back at that door, I look back at those ten years, and at what drove Nigel to make the choice he made. What compelled him – a man who loved life – to end it here, at Dignitas, in Zurich, on 25 April 2017?

2
DEATH'S CALLING CARD

November 2006

Nigel digs the dirt from the grooves of his Callaway five iron with an old tee peg. Three and nine irons, soaking in soapy water in the sink, await the same treatment.

'Big match, Nig?' says Melanie, as she sips her coffee at our battered, pine kitchen table.

Nigel's tongue skids round his mouth like a scooter in a skate park as he says, 'Na. Jushya row wi' ah ki.'

'Pardon?' gags Melanie, coffee splurting down her chin.

He spins around from the sink and attempts to repeat his words, but abandons the effort with an exasperated, 'Ah, fuck it.'

'I think that was "Just a round with our kid,"' I say, ignoring Melanie's alarmed expression and chucking her a tea-towel. I reach for his face. 'You struggling today, love?'

'Yeah,' he says, kissing my hand. 'My tongue feels weird. One minute it's twisting all over the place, the next it's heavy as a brick.'

'What's going on, Nig? asks Melanie.

'Dunno,' he chokes, placing his five iron alongside the sparkling seven in the black and grey Callaway golf bag in the corner, before plunging the nine iron in the sink. 'Can't talk. It's no big deal. Be right tomorrow.'

'But –'

'More coffee Mel?' I blurt. My face performing 'discuss it later' gymnastics as I mouth 'not now.'

'No thanks,' she mutters, getting the message.

Melanie, a younger, striking female version of Nigel, with lavish, raven tresses and bone structure to die for, buries her face in her mug while her troubled, lagoon blue eyes follow her brother's every move. I suspect her motive for her trip from Newcastle is more about her anxiety over the creeping deterioration in Nigel's speech, than it is to update us on her new love and marriage break-up. Melanie frets like a traumatised chimp if your temperature soars one degree above normal, or if you're ten minutes late arriving at her house. Compared to Mel, Florence Nightingale is a meanspirited old witch.

I grab an onion and tray of mince from the fridge and, in a showy pretence of apathy regarding Nigel's speech, chop the onion into tiny chunks.

'What's for tea?' Nigel asks.

'Chilli. I'm making a massive pot.'

'Lovely,' says Mel.

Clubs cleaned, he retrieves his putter and a ball from the bag, takes a pint glass from the wall cupboard and places it on the floor, to act as a hole.

'Bloody hell, serious stuff this. You playing for a tenner?' I say.

'More like twenty.'

I chuck the mince into the pan to brown, stirring as Nigel concentrates on his technique. Chewing his bottom lip, squinting at the target, he strokes the head of the putter towards the ball. If someone happened to graft Nigel's hands onto a musician's wrists, you would have one apoplectic musician. However, you'd be granted a delighted high five from a gorilla. Grapple hook fingers grip the putter as if it's made of butter. It's all about soft hands is golf. I appreciate this as I played – I use the term loosely – back when Nigel and I first met in 1975. I gave up, not without tremendous relief, when juggling kids and work provided me with the perfect excuse to put a halt to the torment. Four hours of stress and humiliation and vomiting in a bush whenever I hit a rotten shot does not make for a fun day out. I now limit such self-imposed misery to the odd round with Nigel, on holiday, where a glass of wine at the halfway house on the ninth, makes it altogether less odious.

Nigel, in comparison, gains as much pleasure from the game as I do pain. He doesn't mind in the least if he has a harrowing round. Why worry if your drive slices across two wrong fairways, when your recovery shots are legendary? Approachable, a true man's man, he's as popular in the pub and rugby club as he is at the golf club. The banter with the blokes both on the course and in the Nineteenth are more important to him than a spanking score.

'Woah! Eat your heart out Tiger.' I applaud as the ball rattles across the tiles and hits the back of the glass. 'The twenty quid is yours methinks.'

'A knocking bet,' he grins.

'Did somebody mention twenty quid?' says Les, bursting into the kitchen. Every member of the family, not to mention the odd burglar, wanders unchecked into our home. Les leans his mismatched clubs in their non branded bag – he's not as dedicated as his brother – against the doorframe. 'Hey, it's that Mel,' he cries, embracing his youngest sis in an exuberant hello.

'Ey up, our kid,' says Nigel. 'Got your losing tackle with you I see.'

Les hesitates before responding, 'You mean winning tackle, mate.'

'Twenty quid says otherwise,' says Nigel.

The concerned, now familiar glance, passes between Les and Melanie and next to me. Les inhales as if to speak further, but the words remain trapped behind pursed lips. It's like the moment you are confronted with a puss-spewing coldsore on someone's chin, and in a split second you choose between, 'What's that awful mess on your face?' or a tactful silence. Les opts for somewhere in between.

'You sound knackered, mate. You up for this?'

'Damn right,' says Nigel, replacing the putter and, his words indistinct and muffled, adds, 'I can't talk today, but I can still thrash you at golf.'

Removing his glasses before tugging the navy jumper, monogrammed with the initials SSCGC (Scarborough South Cliff Golf Club) over his head, he makes a show of smoothing the long since disappeared hair, and performs, as he does whenever he steps out of the shower or a swimming pool, an elaborate flick of the magnificent Elvis quiff that once adorned his handsome head.

'You're such a tit,' laughs Melanie.

He is Bruce Willis in *Die Hard* kind of bald, where, having lost the hair from the top of his head, the only acceptable thing to do is remove the rest of the offending stuff.

'You'll need this mate,' says Les, flinging Nigel his flat tweed cap. 'It's going to rain and you've nowt to protect yer bonce.' Older by two years, Les, much to Nigel's irritation, has retained his hair.

Nigel grins and chucks it back. 'I'll live. It doesn't rain in the Nineteenth. Come on.'

He swings the bulky bag of clean clubs onto his shoulder like it's a feather pillow. He always carries, never bothers with a trolley. It's a macho thing, I reckon.

'See ya later girls,' says Les.

Mel waves them off. 'Play well.'

Nigel adjusts his cap and leans to kiss my cheek. 'Right love, won't be late.'

'Yeah right,' I snigger. They'll be stuck in the Nineteenth for hours. 'Have a nice game.'

As they turn to leave, the door opens and Paula scoots in, carrying a scone-laden tray.

'Hello everybody. I've made scones.'

She places the mountain on the worktop and returns Melanie's welcoming embrace. Nigel and Les offer a hasty 'Hi' and 'Bye' as they shuffle past.

'Not being rude Paula,' says Nigel. 'There's twenty quid at stake.'

'Don't worry. Enjoy.'

'Ooo great, I'm starving,' says Mel, surveying the delights. 'Can I scoff one now?'

'Of course. I've done some herby ciabatta bread to go with the chilli later.'

She's a feeder my sister. Whilst she seldom samples her delicious culinary masterpieces herself, she finds foisting them on others irresistible. Pinned above her range in her, 'I mean business,' cook's kitchen, hangs a tile which reads: 'Lord, if you won't make me skinny, please make my friends fat.' I suspect she doesn't trust the Lord to do the job, so she's embarked on the mission herself.

'Ah lovely, thanks P.'

'There's strawberry jam, and cream as well.'

'Would expect nothing less, Sis.'

'Proper afternoon tea,' says Mel.

'There's no tea on the menu,' says Paula. 'That would be plain daft. I'll pop back up for wine.'

Mel scowls. 'Does wine go with scones?'

'Champagne?' I suggest.

'Perfect. Bubbles. I'll run up and add it to the pile,' says Paula, dashing back upstairs to the flat, which, once upon a time, housed the five bedrooms of our grand Victorian home. When we bought the place in 1990 it was arranged as two flats, the upstairs having a private staircase to the side. We proceeded to throw many thousands of pounds and skip-loads of love into the deserving money pit and restored it to a single dwelling, boasting a magnificent central staircase leading to cavernous, elegant rooms, all festooned with intricate cornices and countless period features.

Years later, when our three kids, Craig, Ellie and Becky, abandoned us to pursue their dreams, whether in a fit of pique for they had left, or the possibility of their reappearance bearing many small children, we threw yet more thousands of pounds at it and, not without considerable heartbreak, tore down that magnificent central staircase. Paula and Tom bought and converted the first floor into a splendid two bed flat and we adapted our own ground floor into a flat of equal grandeur – some would refer to them as apartments, but we're from Yorkshire and a flat is a flat – and, to make up for the loss of five bedrooms, we stuck a knob of a conservatory on the back. I've never got over it.

It did, however, free us of the never-ending, interest-only mortgage. That interest being a whopping 18%.

...

The cork flies from the bottle with a convivial pop. Melanie and Paula hold their flutes aloft as I pour the sparkling champagne from what will no doubt be the first of many bottles.

'Cheers.'

'Mmm. More than respectable,' says Paula, scrutinising the label.

'Plenty more where that came from, girls. I've a garage full of the stuff in readiness for Christmas.'

I lean back in the vintage farmhouse armchair, most often reserved for Nigel, put my feet on the table and prepare to let the welcome bubbles perform their magic. When it comes to hosting drinkers, our table could compete with any pub in the country, and, I shouldn't wonder, Munich's famous Hofbrauhaus. It bears the scars of many sessions, stained to its core from gallons of spilled beer and wine, mutilated by distracted guests digging holes in it with a corkscrew, or Tracey, Nigel's other sister, defluffing those holes with the hooks of her earrings.

It has witnessed joyful gatherings where we revellers sing along whilst Craig belts out well-loved tunes on his keyboard. It held us captive for weeks when planning each minuscule detail of Ellie's and Danny's wedding. This table has thundered with shrieks of raucous laughter, captured and dried waterfalls of tears, guarded and cherished many long held secrets. It has supported dancing feet, snoozing corpses, drunken heads and the odd bare bum, although we don't mention that when Becky's around.

'What the hell's up with our Nig's speech, Julie?' says Mel, with her characteristic boldness. 'It's terrible.'

'He does sound drunk all the time,' adds Paula. 'First thing in the morning's worse.'

I wonder if the two of them have rehearsed this. Plotted an ambush, determined to raise the problem Nigel and I have, not ignored, rather failed to discuss with anybody.

I fill our glasses. 'Yes, I know. His speech is worsening. I managed to convince him to go to the doctor.'

'Oh?' they say, eyebrows shooting up in anticipation.

'What did he say?' says Mel.

'She.'

'OK, what did she say?'

'That's the trouble. She's no idea.'

Paula slams her glass on the table. 'Bloody hell.'

'How come she's no idea?' says Mel, taking a few outraged gulps and a further top up, before continuing. 'So, now what?'

I explain both Nigel's and the doctor's preferred option is to do nothing and see what happens. I suggested consulting a speech therapist.

'Well, it's a start,' says Mel. What does our Nig say?'

'He's humouring me. He's not the slightest bit concerned.'

'How come?'

'He's convinced it's stress. Pressure of work.'

'Stress? Is the business in trouble?' Mel asks.

'No. Couldn't be better. Booming, in fact.'

'Stress?' repeats Paula, 'Seriously?'

'Yes, I know. It's bollocks,' I say, sharing their disbelief, 'I've never known Nig stressed. Ever. And, since when has stress affected anybody's ability to speak?'

We fall silent as we contemplate the connection between stress and speech, whilst Eva Cassidy's haunting timbre fills the room with, *Somewhere Over the Rainbow*. I refill our glasses. We clink. Sip. Sip again. We meet each other's gaze, each worried expression a reflection of the other.

After a moment, Paula takes a deep breath and breaks the silence with, 'Do you think he's had a stroke?'

I jump like she's slapped me across the face and snap, 'Don't be stupid!'

This is unfair, because, as a quality manager of an FE college, my medical knowledge is boundless.

I fail to mention I had been thinking precisely that.

3
BRENDA AND METHUSELAH

November 2006

We arrive at Brenda's compact semi-detached bungalow a few minutes early for our appointment. She's watching for us at the voile-dressed picture window, and opens the door in welcome as we pull onto the driveway.

With the exception of her broad smile, everything about her is petite. I'm surprised, as I had invented a rounder Brenda, with rosy cheeks, grey, shampoo-and-set hair, heavy rimmed glasses, feet wrapped in cosy slippers and a floral pinny tied around an ample waist. Instead, a short silver bob frames a pale oval face. Amber eyes, sparkling with vitality, peer from atop multicoloured specs perched on the end of her angular nose. She's wearing an emerald fitted shift dress and bright red crocs.

'Come in out of the cold,' she insists. 'I'm Brenda. You must be Nigel and Julie.'

We are invited into a tiny porch, housing a pale blue raincoat, one of those transparent birdcage umbrellas and a pair of green wellies. As I make to remove my boots, I stumble against Nigel in the cramped space, which he fills. He's not a bulky man: five foot eight, could stretch to six feet were it not for the bandy legs, of average build and not at all overweight. Indeed, beneath his brown leather jacket, tight-fitting T-shirt and thigh hugging denim jeans, lurks one powerful, musclebound hunk of a bloke, with a body sculptured to perfection from years of physical hard work. But right now, his textbook body needs to vacate Brenda's porch.

'Don't worry,' she says. 'Just give them a brisk rub. Come in both of you. Tea, coffee?'

We opt for tea.

The fruity, tantalising aroma of freshly baked Christmas cake wafts towards us as we follow Brenda into her home.

'Mmm,' I sniff, 'been baking?'

'Yes, I always make my Christmas cake in November. I shouldn't. It'll be gone before December. Cake is one of my many weaknesses I'm afraid.'

'Not surprised. It smells divine.'

Brenda's kitchen, like her, is tidy and tiny. Nigel waits outside in the hall to conserve precious space. By the time the kettle boils, I've concluded Brenda is widowed and lives alone. I must stop making assumptions. Just as Brenda is petite and not round, I insist on fabricating a person's entire life, without a smidgen of evidence. Their abode, the car they drive, choice of wallpaper, state of the garden, will suffice. Therefore, a widow due to a lack of clues portraying a masculine presence. No man's hat and coat in the porch, perhaps as well, as there's no room. No half-read newspaper spread across the table, no garden spade leaning against the shed at the end of the manicured lawn, no photograph on the mantlepiece. I took a sneaky peek into the lounge as we passed. No photographs at all, in fact. Anywhere.

'Cake?' asks Brenda.

We decline, not wishing to share responsibility for its untimely disappearance.

As we observe Brenda arrange a tray with the prettiest porcelain cups I've ever seen, accompanied by matching teapot, sugar bowl and milk jug, I am struck by the beauty of her hands. They are delicate and smooth, belying her obvious age, and her impeccable nails are painted a bright red. It's then I detect the lack of rings on her fingers. No wedding ring. Ah, not a widow, Julie? Blown that theory to hell. A spinster, I decide. No hubby, no kids. She may, in fact, have had three husbands and five kids, yet chooses not to decorate her home with mugshots of her brood. Unlike my kitchen walls, so plastered with portraits it's impossible to stick a finger between the frames.

Why don't I ask?

'How long did you work for the NHS?' I ask, instead, wishing it didn't appear like I was checking her credentials.

As one would expect from a speech therapist, her manner of speech is even and controlled, and she explains she spent twenty years working at Hull Royal Infirmary before moving to the market town of Northallerton, six years ago, to be near her sister, where she has since practised privately. No mention of a husband. I'm tempted to probe further but she interrupts my inept un-Holmes-like deductions by switching the focus onto us, and we are obliged to explain that Nigel owns a scaffolding and a roofing company and I work in a college.

She leads us into the conservatory overlooking the garden and invites Nigel to take a seat at the glass topped and cane legged dining table while I make myself comfortable on the floral sofa at the other side of the room, deftly skirting the fluffy white cat, camouflaged on the sheepskin rug. Our presence is of such trifling interest it doesn't stir. Or, it could be dead.

Porcelain figurines, Lladro, I suspect, of ladies adopting elegant poses line the windowsill. A spinster. Got to be. I bet she has one of those ballerina toilet roll covers.

Brenda hands me a cup of tea. 'Thank you,' I say, clocking once again those red nails and striking red crocs. An image of a ripped toy boy chained to the radiator in her bedroom comes unbidden into my warped mind, along with a plethora of sex toys loitering in her knicker drawer. What the hell is wrong with me?

Brenda offers Nigel an ever so fragile cup and saucer. 'Nigel, tell me what's happening?'

I study Nigel as he takes the cup of tea. No way will his finger fit through that miniature handle. No way. When Nigel's hand's not twirling a scaffold spanner it's clutching a pint of beer. He takes the saucer in one hand and with the thumb and forefinger of the other, he grips the teeny handle of the cup and, twinkling aquamarine eyes reflecting the cornflower blue of his T-shirt, sticks out his pinky. Daft bugger.

'Well, I'm struggling to speak.'

'Suddenly?'

'No. It's been getting worse for a while. Some days my speech is fine, but other days the words are slurred and I sound drunk.'

Apart from the flatness of tone and heavy nasal quality, Nigel's speech today remains comprehensible.

'Have you been involved in an accident? A bang to the head, or any kind of trauma?'

'No. Nothing like that.'

'And this has developed gradually? Not overnight?'

'Yes.'

'OK, Nigel, let's explore what's happening,' says Brenda.

Adjusting her specs, she opens a file and hands him a sheet of paper. She asks him to read aloud the list of words on the page.

'Take your time. There's no hurry.'

Nigel shuffles in the chair and clears his throat. I sense his unease. I recall him telling me how he hated reading aloud at school. At first, he copes well. Individual words present no problem. As he continues to read, he struggles with the plosive consonants such as, 't', 'd', 'k' and 'g,' where the middle and back of the tongue need to become involved in the job. He sounds like a kid reciting tongue twisters with a gobstopper in his mouth. The more he grapples with the words, the more unintelligible it becomes. His strong hands grip the edge of the table as he persists.

We're grateful when Brenda interrupts. 'Rest a moment, while I make a few notes.'

Nigel leans back in his chair and takes a deep breath. 'Bloody hell, what just happened?'

Baffled, I return his gaze. Nigel's speech would never be tested like this: in a continuous stream of sentences. He's not the type to babble or dominate conversations. He speaks with others, not at them, and is content to dip in and out with a well-timed retort, an observation, an anecdote at the most.

'Ready?' says Brenda after a couple of minutes.

'Yes,' he mutters. He's no quitter.

The sentences now are longer and more complex and Nigel stumbles over the phrases like a schoolboy learning to read. An anxious, hesitant beginning soon deteriorates to the point where his speech is incoherent. His shoulders are rigid and hands, balled into tight fists, rub against his thighs with each forced utterance. His distress is difficult to watch, so I try and concentrate on the cat, the figurines, the carpet of fallen leaves in the garden. To no avail. I abandon that idea. Whatever this is, we have it to deal with. I close my eyes and listen.

...

There is an ancient bristlecone pine tree living high in the White Mountains above California. It is close to five thousand years old.

Its name is Methuselah.

Exposed and alone, it rises from the stark, snow-covered earth and stands, wounded but not conquered by centuries of ferocious winds, like a dedicated warrior defending a desolate landscape. Fissures, like rivers of molten copper, encircle the magnificent trunk, bronzed and blackened with age. Twisted by time, it's as if, every thousand years or so, tiring of the view, Methuselah turns and looks the other way. Naked branches, contorted yet graceful, reach out in all directions, captured for eternity in the midst of an exotic dance.

We all know trees can't talk, yet they can speak to you. Methuselah speaks of wisdom, of commitment and endurance. There is melancholy in its tortured branches and both dominance and resignation in the majesty of its trunk.

It has witnessed much: said nothing.

Imagine, if, after five thousand years of profound silence, this particular tree found a voice? You might suppose it would swell from a low rumble emerging from deep within the belly of its powerful trunk. It would draw on the self-assurance borne of longevity, throbbing with intensifying resonance, until a voice, dragged from the tips of every root and branch, echoes across the mountains in a triumphant roar.

Alternatively, it could be a tremulous beginning filled with uncertainty. Its customary confidence vanished in this unfamiliar place. Here is a mouth that neither belongs nor grasps what it's supposed to do. It refuses to open. The lips are pressed as though glued. This mouth is filled with a clumsy and treacherous tongue. It blocks the space. The breath grates in a constricted throat. It commands all its strength and determination to drag the sound from its core. And when, at last, the garbled commotion erupts, it is in anguished gasps. Like the choking cry of someone buried beneath rubble, like gravel scratching against glass. It is a mournful, primeval, alien voice.

That voice is Nigel's.

...

He shoves the papers across the table. We gape at each other. For the second time in an hour we're grateful to Brenda as she takes charge.

'That's fine, Nigel, we're all finished.' She pats him on the shoulder before gathering the papers. 'Well done.'

Nigel grimaces at the 'well done,' perhaps conscious his level of attainment is unworthy of congratulations. Like the kid who comes in hours after the rest of the pack in the cross-country race, the one who tries his best, unlike those other stragglers guilty of hiding in the woods, smoking with their mates and lobbing stones in the lake. He is the one who is rewarded with a patronising pat on the head for simply taking part. That's not Nigel.

He snatches his jacket from the back of the chair, gripping it in both hands as if intent on tearing it to shreds. 'My bloody tongue doesn't belong to me.'

'Yes, it's very strange. Quite the mystery,' acknowledges Brenda, managing her patient's frustrations with calm assurance, smiling as she places her hand on Nigel's arm. Nigel exhales with a whoosh, his shoulders drop as he relaxes a little. He takes the car keys from the pocket and tucks the jacket under his arm.

'I'll write the report today and it will be in the post to you tomorrow.'

Post? Haven't you heard of email? Not famous for my patience and unable to wait for the report, I ask, 'What is it, do you think?'

'Well,' she says, 'I recognise the condition, but not the cause.'

'Condition?' echoes Nigel.

'Dysarthria. Often referred to as "hot potato speech." Speaking as though a hot potato is wedged in your mouth.'

Perfect. That's it. I make a mental note to jump straight on the net once we're home.

'Treatment?' asks Nigel.

I wonder if today's encounter means my husband will utter no more than one-word sentences from now on.

'Until the cause is established, we can't determine the treatment.'

'What do you suggest we do next?' I say, anxious to be doing something.

'I recommend you consult a neurologist,' she says, and, as if I'm not sufficiently alarmed by today's events, adds, 'Soon.'

The consultation over, we thank Brenda for her time and promise to keep her updated.

Nigel slides the car out of Brenda's drive onto the road. Never one to be pissed off for long, he leans towards me, crow's feet creasing beneath sparkling eyes and says, 'Pub?'

4

TESTS, TESTS AND MORE TESTS

November 2006 – February 2007

After all these years of believing my macho husband invincible, it turns out he's as conquerable as Goliath.

First, the network of veins contained within those magnificent arms are mean. A tad unfortunate, given the requirement to fill the equivalent of many buckets with blood. The purpose of which is unclear.

'Tests,' we are told.

'What are they testing for?' asks Nigel, examining the needle as it is inserted, for a third time, into a shy looking vein. The persistent tapping to coax it isn't working.

'Oh, you know, lots of things, I expect,' says the cheery nurse named Diane, her expression betraying nothing.

Nigel accepts the dismissal without challenge. 'Right.'
I bet he's more interested in where she's from. A characteristic he shares with his dad, Ron and sister Tracey. Two seconds after meeting someone the compulsion to ask overwhelms them.

'At last,' she says, the vein submitting.

'Where're you from?'

There.

'York, born and bred. You?' she says, the tube now full.

'Bradford –'

Unable to contain myself, I interrupt with, 'What are they testing for. Specifically?'

'Oh, nothing to worry your head about,' she says, addressing me like I'm a child. She presses a snippet of cotton wool to the pinprick in Nigel's arm and tapes over it. 'This and that, you know.'

No, I don't know.

'They know what they're doing in the lab,' she continues. 'There, all done.'

Well, that's cleared that up. As long as they know, eh?

Second, he is claustrophobic. Discovered when a violent and unexpected panic attack overwhelmed him as the medical team attempted an MRI scan. Again, like the bloodletting, the reason for the MRI remains a mystery.

'Expect a barrage of tests,' said the neurologist at Nigel's first appointment. Didn't mention the 'what' and the 'why.'

We're paying, remember.

Claustrophobia is one of those conditions you're unaware of until you find yourself stuck in a lift, trapped in a hole, or sucked into a scanner. I suppose the horror Nigel has at the prospect of potholing or working down a mine, should have provided a clue to his potential susceptibility. As it is, he hit upon a career which suits his temperament, where claustrophobic-inducing situations are rare. His life is spent swinging on scaffolding structures from tube to tube with the confidence and agility of a gibbon on the run, at heights where Fred Dibnah would break into a sweat. His work-places are motorway bridges, high-rise tower blocks, churches, cathedrals, roller coasters and the odd castle. Anything involving going up before coming down is okay with Nigel – parachuting, bungee jumping and gliding – all enjoyed as a result of birthday gifts aiming for something a dash more adventurous than a pair of socks and Jean Paul Gaultier aftershave.

Anyway, here we are again, driving along the A64 to York Hospital, for a second attempt at the MRI, and we still can't fathom why we're doing it. On this occasion though, he has reinforcements. He has me, a stock of Lorazapam tablets and Bupa Bear. The teddy is poised in the back seat, exuding comfort and courage, as is his role in life. Bupa Bear, a reward from the staff of Scarborough's Bupa hospital, for eight year old Ellie's bravery following an operation on her nose. Since then, he's been right up there with chicken soup and *Muppet Babies* videos, a vital member of the nursing team, tackling each childhood illness that dares to come along. Ellie shared Bupa's healing abilities with her siblings, including older brother Craig, who, though he forbade the teddy to sleep on his pillow, would at least permit him to share the bottom of the bed. So, hearing of her dad's panic attack, she popped Bupa Bear in the post without delay, hoping his superpowers would extend to carrying her dad into that MRI scanner.

Nigel shovels another Lorazapam in his mouth. 'How many of those did the doctor say you should take?'

'Two.'

'How many have you taken?'

'Three. Maybe four.'

I stop myself from saying, 'Is that wise?' and keep my mouth shut. We don't need a row now. The interior of our Mondeo is a cauldron of simmering apprehension, threatening to boil over as every mile delivers us closer to the hospital.

Nigel reclines the passenger seat as far as it will allow. His eyes are squeezed as shut as the 'see no evil' monkey's, and the fan of wrinkles carved in his skin is more prominent than usual. Jaw clenched, fists stuffed into the pockets of his leather jacket, as if feigning sleep to avoid discussion. It's not working. I can tell he's far from sleep by the way he keeps clearing his throat and shuffling in his seat. Come on Nig, my fearless, unconquerable husband, you're in there somewhere. You've never lost a fight or run away from anything in your life. Perhaps the numbing effect of the Lorazapam has provoked his sombre mood. It's not like him. Nigel finds hilarity even in tragic circumstances and digs up a joke – however tasteless – from the depths of a mass grave. But there is to be no joking today.

I glimpse Bupa in the rear view mirror. Hope you've brought bucket loads of courage, cuddly bear. Maybe we should've enlisted the additional help of Buffy the Vampire Slayer to vanquish Nigel's fiends.

We reach the hospital.

'Shall I take Bupa along?' I say, grabbing the bear from the back seat. I'm joking, of course. How ridiculous would a bloke like Nigel look, snuggling a teddy? No matter how cute.

I am rewarded with a hint of a smile. He takes the bear from me and strokes its furry brown head before tossing poor Bupa over the seat into the back. He grasps my hand and raises it to his lips to kiss it. 'Love you,' he says.

'Love you too.'

'Come on. I can do this.'

'You can do anything,' I acknowledge, leaning into the back to perch Bupa Bear upright. 'Sorry,' I whisper.

It's a short, Lorazapam-induced, totter to the waiting room, where Nigel swallows yet another tablet.

It's time. I take his arm, to steady him, as we are led into an area with curtained cubicles. He is instructed to undress, don a cotton gown and remove his watch. From here, we are ushered into the scanning room, or, depending on your viewpoint, chamber of horrors. Two nurses, both built like nightclub door supervisors, guard the instrument of torture.

'Back for another shot at it, Mr Casson?' says a nurse with greying hair scraped so visciously into a bun on top of her head, her eyebrows are yanked halfway up her forehead. 'Let's have you.'

Her menacing voice grates like her face. Too long in the job I suspect. Run out of patience with patients. Nigel grunts and shuffles towards the scanner.

'Come on, Mr Casson, we'll look after you,' says the younger nurse, opening her arms as if to enfold Nigel within them. 'We'll manage this time. We've arranged for some relaxing music to play while you're in there.'

Angela, I note from her badge, pats the patient's table like it's Santa's knee. 'Up you pop.'

Alright Ange, he's fifty-two, not six.

Nigel moves like a diver in lead boots. Beads of sweat dampen his brow and his breath comes in ragged bursts. Jangling, nasal grunts, unrecognisable as words, erupt from his mouth. He could be protesting, begging for mercy, or telling a joke. He clambers onto the table like he weighs thirty stone.

'Come on now,' says the bun, as he rests his head on a piece of moulded plastic.

Angela fastens a mask-like contraption over his face and locks it in place. 'Try and relax, we've got you. Lie still and listen to the music. Think happy thoughts.'

That's all he needs. His head in a box. I grab his hand. He closes his eyes. They crank the thing up.

'It's OK,' I whisper.

He opens his eyes and regards me through the screen. No it's not, they say. He might as well be pizza dough about to be rammed into a burning hot oven.

It takes all his courage, and he has loads of it, to command his body to cease its trembling and calm his breathing. I grip his hand as he slides into the scanner until I'm forced to let go. This is the first time Nigel's vulnerabilty has surfaced. The first time I've witnessed his fear.

Wish I'd brought Bupa Bear in with us now.

...

Nigel stands facing the back wall of a compact examination room, naked except for his Calvin Klein, low-rise undies. Doctor Afik Khan, impossible to comprehend how he's acquired doctor status, despite the neat moustache and closely trimmed beard, as there's no way he's older than fifteen, stands behind him. Young, handsome and a doctor. His parents must be tickled pink.

'Place your hands on your hips please,' he says.

Nigel obeys.

Doctor Khan cups his chin in one hand, cups his elbow with the other and appraises Nigel's body in silence. Minutes pass. Then some more. I study the doctor as he gawps at Nigel, from my spot in the corner of the room. We are exceptionally still. It's like the music has stopped in a game of 'statues' and the host has buggered off with the CD player without telling the rest of us the party is over.

What is he expecting to see? I muse, and fail to ask, as per.

Doctor Khan instructs Nigel to spin around to face him, whereupon he ogles some more. He studies Nigel's body like he's pondering the magnificence of Michelangelo's David.

Yes, gorgeous isn't he? I'm inclined to remark, as I too admire that familiar toned torso, those well-developed biceps, those awesome, uber strong thighs. As usual, I keep my mouth shut. This is bloody creepy. Nigel could be a rent boy parading before punters. I swivel on the chair so I can see his face and discover he isn't the slightest bit perturbed. He's biting his bottom lip to imprison the threatening guffaw and he winks at me, the devil himself dancing in his eyes.

Please don't ask him to pace up and down. I envisage him strutting his stuff, hands on hips, wriggling his bum like he's playing the lead in *The Full Monty*. The doctor doesn't ask. He twists away from Nigel and orders him to climb onto the examination table for the next stage in the procedure. The procedure, we are informed, is known as electromyography, or EMG test. It's something to do with muscles and nerves.

'Where're you from,' asks Nigel. Surprise, surprise.

'Harrogate.'

'Great town,' he says, proceeding to name the buildings and streets upon which he has erected scaffolding, whilst the doctor, oblivious to Nigel's anecdotes, places sensors and electrodes on his skin.

'Brilliant golf course, too,' Nigel persists. 'I nearly had a hole in one on the fourth, or was it the fifth?'

Attractive young man, with proud parents, he may be, but Doctor Kahn wouldn't trouble first place in a bedside manner contest.

Next, as if punishment for the lack of any kind of performance from the lengthy observation of that superb anatomy, thirty painful minutes pass as the doctor punches long needles deep into the offending muscles of Nigel's arms, legs, back and throat. It takes less than a minute to shut Nigel up. Whatever is taking place inside those muscles is translated through the electrodes and needles into graphs on the computer screen and Doctor Khan, thorough and in no hurry, spends several minutes analysing the data before him.

'Mmm. Inconclusive,' he says at last. 'Come back in a month and we'll do it again.'

Brilliant. Can't wait.

...

We're in an agreeable room at the private Nuffield hospital in York. Nigel is in bed, gowned and ready for surgery. Les is stationed at one side of the bed, I'm at the other. The surgeon, Mr Field, has made a mark on Nigel's thigh muscle from where he will take the biopsy. He takes the time to explain in detail – this happens when you're a private patient – how long the procedure will take and when we'll be allowed home.

'They'll be along to collect you shortly,' he says.

'Don't call me shortly,' jokes Nigel, a retort he never fails to employ when presented with the opportunity.

Mr Field chuckles politely, something else that happens when you're a private patient. He addresses the room. 'He'll be gone around an hour.'

'I'll wait here, mate. Read the paper,' says Les, who's come along to do the driving home. Or, he's nothing better to do today. The two of them will no doubt call for a pint back in Scarborough.

'I'll pop to Tesco's, do a massive shop,' I say, keen to take advantage of the superior and gigantic store at nearby Clifton Moor.

'I'll have mi' leg off then,' says Nigel, grinning.

Another polite snicker as Mr Field leaves the room with, 'The results of the tests will be with your neurologist by the end of next week.'

'Right,' I say. Tests for what? I wonder. And obviously, I don't ask.

5

THE END OF 'NORMAL'

10 February 2007

The stunning renovation of a sixties, three-bed suburban semi in Shipley fails to stun me. In truth, I couldn't give a shit. Snapping the *House Beautiful* magazine shut, I fling it on the beech coffee table with unwarranted irritation. Could do with some stunning renovation round here, if you ask me. Must hospital reception areas be limited to the colours pink and green? Has some edict been imposed on such establishments? Three months of wilting in one wishy-washy waiting room after another. The tired décor of this one stares back at me. Pastel pink walls bearing cockeyed pictures of white lilies, pale green carpet and impractical pink chairs, rubbed grey by hundreds of backsides. Even the lush umbrella plant in the corner fails to lift the insipid palette. Colours that make you feel ill when you're not. I expect better from a private hospital.

'How much longer do you suppose?' I spit, not caring if the receptionist hears me. She does. The thirty-something attractive brunette behind the desk glances up and throws me an indulgent smile. The kind of smile you plaster on your face when hoping to deter a toddler from having a tantrum.

'Mr Harrop won't be long,' she says. 'You're next. He knows you're here.'

I lower my gaze in shame. I would shove me to the bottom of the list if I had her job.

'Calm down, we've just arrived,' says Nigel. 'We'll drive into York after and grab a bite. I might as well pick up the accounts from John's, while we're here. And there's a decent pub near his office.'

Mollified by the thought of lunch and a glass of wine, I slouch in my pink chair and shut up. I like York. It's such a vibrant, enchanting city, bursting with history and culture, a joy to walk round with scores of impressive eateries and a gazillion pubs, all of which claim to be the oldest and most haunted in the city. There are also many shops, if you happen to be into shopping, which I'm not.

Nigel uses the time to sketch the scaffolding framework needed for the job he measured up on route.

'Do you suppose we'll get the test results today?' I ask, unable to keep quiet for long.

He drags his attention away from his jottings and fixes me with a blank gaze. 'Maybe. Dunno. We'll see, eh?'

He resumes the task of listing the required scaffold poles: five foots, ten foots, twenty-ones. Some time ago the back of a fag packet served admirably as his office. Way back in 1984, when we bade farewell to the West Yorkshire town of Cleckheaton and chugged along the A64 towards Scarborough, like hillbillies setting off on holiday. Me, the kids and all our possessions, crammed in the back of a battered old Transit van on the way to our new home: an imposing block of thirteen holiday flats on Scarborough's South Cliff.

My dad came up with the idea of investing in a single holiday flat to rent out to cover its mortgage. It took no more than a couple of property viewings for Nigel to discover a significant proportion of Scarborough's buildings are old, tall and difficult to access. Combined with the advertisement of a businessman in the local yellow pages, whose tagline boasted, 'Scarborough's *only* scaffolder,' the acorn became an oak tree.

Mum and Dad, Paula and her then husband Joe, were all keen to be part of the adventure, and within months we had sold our properties, combined resources for the deposit and secured the flats. With Mum and Paula's help, I would manage the flats, the income from which would pay the mortgage and bills. Nigel borrowed a terrifying two thousand pounds to buy the scaffolding needed to establish his company. Dad – a painter and decorator – declared himself more than happy to enliven the décor of Scarborough's homes rather than those of Halifax. Paula was confident she would find work, and certain her husband, executive of I'm not sure what, would continue endlessly travelling the country.

Business networking, in those days, took place in pubs and clubs. Within weeks, Nigel, already a member of the South Cliff Golf Club and Scarborough Rugby Club, made it his mission to visit the full gamut of pubs in the town, immersed in his research, determined to find drinkers in need of the services of a new scaffolding company. He met Glyn, a local window cleaner, soon to become Nigel's business partner. Given the brutal effect of salty sea air on glass, window cleaning in Scarborough is a lucrative occupation, and in those first few months Nigel and Glyn helped each other out by juggling window cleaning and scaffolding.

Meanwhile, me and the kids adapted to our new lives. Craig, never comfortable until his surroundings are conquered, carried out the equivalent of the 'knowledge' on his bike, cycling up and down the maze of streets, parks and pathways in the town until he considered himself at home. Ellie, a happy child, remained in a perpetual state of excitement because we lived a ten-minute walk from the beach, and Becky, a mere baby, became accustomed to having a busy and distracted mother and, disturbingly often, no cot to sleep in, whenever the flats' supply couldn't meet demand.

The whims and concerns of the guests consumed my life. A shortage of teaspoons, a loose pan handle, a cracked plate. Nothing worried our guests more than the white furry element in their flat's kettle. They'd stand at my door, brandishing the offending object, something approaching genuine fear on their faces, and point at the poisonous substance lurking inside.

'It's harmless,' I would explain. 'Caused by Scarborough's hard water.'

Waste of breath. They never believed me. In the end, I swapped my own kettle for theirs. I was getting through three kettles a week by the end of month two.

We lived in that multi-generational home for four years without having a single row. But our growing children needed more independent space, and I had secured a part-time teaching job at the local FE College. Also, I had become bored of the kettle wars. Nigel's business was thriving and the window-cleaning had long since been abandoned.

Now, twenty-five years on, as many men work for them. Some of the town's iconic architecture: the Grand Hotel, the Spa Complex, Valley Bridge, Spa Bridge, and also the Castle, all propped up, at some point, by DNC Scaffolding, without which, I'm certain, the town would slip into the sea. Along the way Nigel and Glyn formed a roofing company to complement the scaffolding business, bought property via their holding company and acquired premises for the storage, hire and sale of scaffolding, roofing and general building equipment. That two thousand pounds and those few pints paid off.

...

'We'll see,' I ponder, dragging my thoughts back to the present. Reminds me of how I'd placate our nagging kids. Be quiet now and bugger off and play is the accurate translation.

I reach for another magazine but hesitate before picking it up. I spot the receptionist looking at us. I'm sure she recognises us, as this is our third appointment. I ignore her and focus on the door we first entered three months since, clutching Brenda's report.

'Dr Peter Harrop. Neurologist,' reads the sign.

Maybe Nigel's right. Maybe it is nothing more than stress. If so, is it necessary to carry out so many blood tests? Should you be expected to endure an MRI scan to determine your stress level? Is there some indicator on your brain that glows red when you're sucked into the tube? Is there any need to endure the pain of electromyography and nerve conduction tests? Twice? And, how could it be normal practice to perform a biopsy on a chunk of your thigh muscle in order to examine it for what? Stress? Stress, my arse.

The door opens and Peter Harrop appears. I leap to my feet. At last. We've been waiting all of seven minutes.

'David. Hello again. Come in, come in. Good to see you.'

For a second I'm confused, I thought we were next. And now Nigel is shaking the neurologist's hand like he's an old mate. Such a mate Nigel hasn't told him his name. I scurry on behind, cursing my husband's parents who gave him the forenames of David Nigel, and thereafter referred to him solely as Nig. What possessed them?

Perhaps they baulked at the name David as soon as they registered it? In those days, maybe they worried Nigel sounded posh? It's feasible, back in the fifties. Up north anyway. Perchance they feared such a label might encourage kids called Gav, Jack or Mick to beat him up? Who knows? So Nig (rhymes with pig) was it. The name 'Nig' is restricted to family now, to others, he's Nige or Nigel. In official circumstances, however, he is always referred to as David. He never tells these professionals his preferred name. It amuses him. It annoys the hell out of me.

So, here I am, sitting next to some bloke called David, before a grand walnut desk. The bulky desk dominates this poky, white, functional room. There's an examination table against the left wall, a tiny sink and four-drawer filing cabinet next to it. Framed certificates share the wall behind the desk with a window, overlooking the car park.

'Now, David, how are you?'

Peter's a congenial chap, fortyish, short, cropped black hair, which fails to disguise approaching baldness. Intelligent eyes, the colour of smoke, regard Nigel with a relaxed, confident air. As you might expect, at seventy-five quid a consultation.

'How's your dad?' says Nigel.

What? Didn't see that coming. How has Nigel met this guy's dad?

'Oh. You know my dad?'

'Well, for a chat over a pint, that's all. He drinks in the Highlander doesn't he? Unusual name "Harrop." I called in there the other week and I asked if he knew you.'

'Right,' says Peter. 'Yes, thank you, he's fine. Although, I've not visited him for a few weeks. I don't often venture to Scarborough.'

'You from Scarborough?'

I struggle to keep my groan inaudible and glance to the heavens for release. However, the gods are busy.

'No, Hull originally. Dad moved to Scarborough when he retired. I live in York now. Anyway,' he says, reverting to the reason why we're in his office. 'How are you?'

He studies Nigel's face with genuine concern and acknowledges me with a blink. I blink back, a smudge of a smile threatens, before I abandon the effort and concentrate on Nigel.

'Any developments?' he says.

'No, I feel fine. It's just this speech. I sound pissed all the time. Which, I am, a lot, but not at eight in the morning. It's a bugger for business.'

'OK, let's examine you again shall we? Sit on the examination table please.'

And once again, like the last visit, Nigel climbs on the bed and follows Peter's instructions to push hard against his shoulder with one leg, then the other. Arms next. Nigel holds out his right arm for Peter to push down on it. It doesn't budge.

'Three of us could swing on that before it gives way.'

We project a polite titter at the humour. It's true, though. Popeye would be jealous of Nigel's muscles.

'And the left.'

To our complete surprise, Nigel's left arm gives way under pressure. That's a change. How odd.

'Have you spotted any weakening in this arm?' Peter asks.

'Maybe after lifting six pints.'

Forever joking. I glare through narrowed eyes at his cheeky, grinning face.

Peter sidesteps the joke and remains focused on the task. 'So, no?'

'No, nothing,' says Nigel, matching Peter's tone.

'Very well.' Peter returns to his seat. 'Stick out your tongue please. And leave it out for as long as you can manage. Alert me if it becomes uncomfortable.' He studies his computer screen, leaving Nigel to follow his instructions.

Nigel sticks out his tongue. A minute passes. It's not possible to look anything other than ridiculous when your tongue is dangling from your mouth, like a panting dog. Nigel grasps the edge of the examination table and swings his legs to and fro as if stuck for something to do.

I can't watch this. I stare at the window instead. The pale blue curtain is grubby and one of the hooks has detached itself from the rail. Seems a bit cheap for Nuffield. Nigel gags, struggling to contain the saliva pooling in his mouth. I fix my gaze on the wall. His drooling should be his alone.

After two torturous minutes, Nigel can stand no more. He coughs, swallows, wipes his mouth with a fist and jumps down from the table. If anything can remove the smile from his face, then this is it.

Peter beckons him back to his seat.

I'm tempted to ask, 'Cat got your tongue?' but a new melancholy hangs in the air and I resist. Peter stares at the screen as though hypnotised. What's he's reading? I tut as a nugget of impatience forms. Must be the test results. Has to be. What's the outcome? Will he tell us in a minute? He will. Of course he will. We're paying after all.

The silence drags on. I glare at Nigel, willing him to say something. Ask the question for God's sake. He ignores me. Should I ask? Is it my place? No, it should be Nigel. I remain quiet so as not to disturb the important fellow behind the desk. I've always deferred to authority: doctors, lawyers, teachers and the like. Today, I hate myself for it.

I cross and re-cross my legs. I reach into my handbag and check for messages on my phone. Three. 'What did he say?' from Craig, 'Any news?' from Ellie. 'How's Dad?' from Becky. I tap Nigel's arm with my phone and show him the messages. 'Right,' he says, stifling a yawn.

I make a massive deal of reading the certificates on the walls behind the desk. How long does it take to become a neurologist? What makes a person choose that particular specialism? Where did he study? Why do I care?

At last, Peter looks away from his computer and leans back in his chair. 'Prepare yourself David, for another barrage of tests.'

'What? More tests?' I snap, as agitation overcomes politeness, 'You said that last time.'

'Why?' says Nigel, finally getting involved. 'What more could there be? What are the results of the others?'

Peter takes a deep breath and adopts a 'let me explain' pose. He leans forward across his magnificent desk, minimising the space between us.

'The tests we've carried out so far, are concerned with elimination.'

Nigel and I confirm our understanding with a nod. Our faces say, 'Go on.'

'I suspect this has been creeping up on you for some time. Picture a cruise liner on the horizon. A dot, barely visible, so distant it's difficult to discern, although you can see something is there. Not until it comes closer does it reveal what it is. These tests tell us what it is not.'

'I see,' says Nigel.

I see too. But I'm not having it. Oh no you don't. No way is today's appointment ending here. No way. You must have an inkling by now. Even I have my suspicions. I've read all there is to read on dysarthria and its causes. There's no way you're clueless, not if those certificates pasted on these walls belong to you.

And so I force him to tell us. 'But what do think it could be? Have you any idea?'

Of course he has. It's written all over his face. His eyes locks with mine, flick to Nigel, then back to me.

'You've asked,' he starts. It's evident from his expression he wishes I hadn't. 'So I must tell you.'

Peter turns to Nigel. My breath locks in my throat. Until now it never occurred to me Nigel might not wish to be told. How could I be so stupid? Has Nigel scoured the net? Drawn similar grim conclusions as I? Chosen to ignore it? Totally absorbed in my own feelings, I'm foisting this on him. I long to yell, 'No, no. Don't tell us, not today.' Too late. Ashamed, I reach for Nigel's hand. He enfolds mine in his and squeezes. We listen, as the neurologist tells us he suspects Nigel has motor neurone disease.

Frozen in the moment, there is the longest pause. I knew it. I see it, itemised in bold, blunt text, like a shopping list of horrors, on my computer screen: the causes of dysarthria. And right there at the top, occupying the number one slot, is motor neurone disease. I convinced myself it couldn't be that. I dismissed it as impossible. It couldn't be. Nigel had something else from that list, something not as atrocious.

'What's that?' says Nigel. A puzzled, but unconcerned expression on his face. I tighten my grip on his hand. He hasn't heard of it. He doesn't know what it is.

The doctor clears his throat. 'This is a disease where the motor neurones, the part of the brain that controls muscle movement, slowly stop working. The cause is unknown. The condition is life-limiting and there is no cure.'

Nigel absorbs the words. He doesn't move, his face remains impassive. All I heard was 'life-limiting' and 'no cure.' I dig my nails into his hand.

'How long have I got?' he asks, coming straight to the point.

'Progression may be slow, or rapid, there is no way of predicting it.'

'How long?'

'Three to five years.'

Nigel draws a long, slow breath. 'Right,' he utters.

Then, like he has diagnosed little more than a cold, Peter asks Nigel if he would be willing to meet one of the country's leading professors on this disease, to confirm his diagnosis. Nigel agrees without hesitation.

'I'll write a prescription for Riluzole now. The only medication available for MND. It prolongs life by two, possibly three months.'

Awesome.

We listen, numb, as he tells us he will now contact Nigel's GP and all appropriate health professionals. We should expect to hear from a physiotherapist, occupational therapist, speech therapist and someone from St Catherine's Hospice. The hospice? That's for dying people. Look at him, my invincible husband, so strong, so fit. No way he's dying. And yet it is clear, however many doctors, therapists and professors are involved from this point on, this is ending one way and one way only. Nigel is going to die.

Moments like this are not at all what you imagine. There is no warning. No darkening sky, no rumble of thunder. The sky is still blue and the sun still shines. Your heart doesn't miss a beat and the world doesn't hold its breath. There is a stark ordinariness. Everything remains exactly the same as it was a moment before. The curtain at the window is still grubby, one of its hooks detached from the rail. The desk is still cumbersome and the window still overlooks the car park where people meander towards their vehicles contemplating what to pick up for tea. The doctor's hairline is still receding, and his dad will still drink in the Highlander.

Nothing has changed. And yet, for us, everything has changed. Nothing will ever be the same again.

6
LIFE WITH MND BEGINS

'Thank you,' says Nigel, shaking Peter Harrop's hand as we leave his office.

'Best of luck,' says Peter, the smile on his lips not reaching his eyes. We won't be here again. There's no point.

Nigel drives, as planned, to the accountant's premises at Peasholme Green, two minutes from York's city centre. Following such news, should we be doing something else? And what would that be? What are you supposed to do when told you're dying? There are no instructions, no guidelines to prepare you for moments like this, no recognised conventions to lead you through steps one, two and three. Sticking to the plan, carrying on as though nothing extraordinary has taken place, feels like the best thing to do.

We pull up outside John's office and claim the last parking space. 'Won't be long,' Nigel says, leaping from the car, 'I'll grab the accounts and say a quick hello.'

I lean back in my seat and close my eyes. How will such a tête-à tête pan out? I wonder.

'Hello Nigel, how are you?'

'Hi John, I'm fine, well, I feel fine, but I'm dying. Not sure how long I've got left. We'd better set a date in the diary for a meeting, discuss what to do.'

A minute later the car door opens. Nigel climbs in and places the box file containing the accounts of another successful year on the back seat. Another year of recounting the growth and profits which will inform the coming year's strategies. Which aspect of the business to expand? Which, if any, to contract? How to ensure tax efficiency? Should they take on more scaffolders or roofers, or both? Will profits increase, or just workload? Typical, end of year analysis. It doesn't matter a damn anymore.

'Well?' I say, scrutinising his expressionless face.

'He's not there. Let's grab a drink. The Black Swan is round the corner.'

The aged timber framed façade of the Black Swan Inn transports us to medieval times before we walk through its slanted front door, and make our way along a creaking oak corridor to the bar at the back. It smells of soot, pub grub and beer. Flames, dancing in the giant open fireplace, are reflected in round copper-topped tables. The crackling fire, along with the dark wood panelling lining the walls, the low, beamed ceiling and crooked, leaded windows conspire to embrace us in the warmest of welcomes. The majority of tables are filled with occupants speaking in hushed tones. It's a calming place, the kind of place where you close your eyes, exhale a long slow breath and trust that now, cocooned within the safety of this soothing room, everything will be OK. How I wish that were true.

There's one table free, in a gloomy corner, the farthest from the fire. It's perfect. Nigel collects the drinks from the bar and we sip, in silence, staring into the room. It occurs to me we must resemble one of those married couples who have run out of things to say. Not that our fellow drinkers appear concerned with anything other than their own lives. A pair of young Asian tourists are peering into the LCD screens of their respective cameras, engrossed in the review of one another's photography. Two tubby, middle-aged men sink their pints of real ale at record speed. Judging by the high fives and jocular arm punching they appear to be recounting past adventures. On a normal day I would ponder the topic of their conversation and contemplate the countries on the young tourists' itinerary. But today is not normal, and other people's stories must wait.

Nigel stares at his pint. Disbelief swims in his eyes. My glass of pinot grigio grows warm in my hand. The incomparable aroma of steak and kidney pie wafts towards us as a waitress hurries by on her way to the dining room.

'Do you fancy some food?' says Nigel.

'No thanks,' I groan. My earlier anticipation of a delicious lunch has now vanished. I couldn't eat a thing. The lump in my throat is choking me. I'm not sure I trust myself to speak. I'm nervous, shy. How ridiculous? Together for thirty-two years and I can't summon the words to comfort my husband following the worst possible news. I mustn't keep from him the fact that I had my suspicions. My Catholic upbringing demands confession. In a tremulous voice, I ask, 'Did you have any idea what the doctor might say?'

Nigel swigs a mouthful of beer. 'No. None at all. Why?'

'You hadn't searched the net?'

'No. Had you?'

'Yes,' I swallow. 'After we'd seen Brenda. I investigated the reasons for dysarthria.'

'And?'

'It's a long list.'

'Motor neurone disease on it?' he asks, in a patient, gentle way, as if sensing my discomfort.

'Yes,' I say, like I'm admitting to nicking a tenner from my mum's purse. 'But I refused to believe it could be MND, I convinced myself it must be something else.'

Nigel reaches for me and pulls me into his arms, cradling me there.

'You poor thing,' he whispers. 'Why didn't you tell me?'

'I didn't want you to be worried.'

'So, you worried all this time on your own?' he says and, as he kisses the tears trapped in my lashes, I'm reminded of how much I love this man.

'I'm sorry,' I say, the weight of my sorrow crushing me from the inside out.

'Don't be. It doesn't matter. It wouldn't make any difference, would it?'

'I can't lose you,' I say, my voice breaking, 'I love you.'

Nigel brushes away a tear from my cheek with his thumb. The tender gesture prompts more. I press my face into his chest, biting hard on my bottom lip to prevent me from opening my despicable mouth again. When did I become the focus of attention? I should be the one comforting him, not the other way around. This isn't me losing Nigel, it's him losing his life. His bittersweet smile pierces my heart as he raises my face to his and kisses the end of my nose.

'I love you too. We'll be okay,' he whispers. 'We'll survive this.' He stops, laughs and swigs another few mouthfuls of beer.

'What?'

'That's not true, is it? I won't survive this.'

I smile in spite of how unfunny the moment is. 'No.'

'But we'll be fine,' he says. 'You and me. We'll cope.'

'You think?'

'Yes I do.'

I marvel at how calm he is. How controlled. I stare at my glass of wine. What will we be required to cope with? Are we armed with the strength we're going to need? The courage? I'm standing at one end of a collapsed bridge, striving to picture the other side of this expanse of infinite darkness. Instinctively, I know I must move from here to there. I must somehow conquer that void. The life we know is finished. It slammed to a stop an hour ago. To embrace the next, this strange, frightening new life, I must find the courage to step into the unknown. Has Nigel already taken that step? Does the clenching and unclenching of his jaw signal that he's preparing to take this thing on? Preparing to fight?

'Come on, we'd better go,' he says, downing his pint.

Reluctant to leave this soothing refuge, I finish the dregs of my warm wine and follow him to the car park to face the cold, stark, new reality of our future.

The car phone is ringing. It's Craig.

'Don't answer it.' I gasp. We've not discussed what to say to the kids. Too late, Nigel has already pressed answer.

'Hi Craig.'

'How'd it go?'

'More tests.'

'Bloody hell. More?'

'Yeah.'

'What are they testing for?'

'Dunno. Eliminating stuff. This 'n' that. No big deal.'

'Mmm.' He sounds unconvinced. 'Oh well. What you doing when you're back? You off to the pub?'

'Yes, setting off now. We'll call at the Indigo for one.'

One?

'Right, catch you tomorrow.'

By misleading Craig, Nigel has at least bought us some time. So, tomorrow it is. Everyone will receive the news tomorrow. I decide the kids must know before anybody else. I don't know why. Is there such a protocol? Does it matter?

'How are we going to tell them? The kids?' I ask.

'We tell them straight. There's no other way. Dressing it up won't help.'

No surprise there either. Nigel is a practical, candid man. Nobody is ever left doubting his intentions. There is nothing ambiguous about him; a characteristic as infuriating as it is endearing.

'Yes I know, I wish we could do it face-to-face, that's all.' This is one of those times when we should all be ensconced around our battered old kitchen table, supporting one another, giving each other strength.

'Not possible.'

He doesn't need to say it, I know it's impossible. The last time we were together was New Year's Eve. With Danny's army career and Becky in the RAF, we're lucky they're even in the same country. At least Craig and his family live in Scarborough.

'We'll ring them tomorrow. So they'll hear it from us.'

He's right of course. I close my eyes and rest my head against the seat.

'Don't worry, they're not made of glass.'

No. No they're not. They're far more fragile than that. If I'm honest, it's not the act of breaking the news that is worrying me the most, it's the news itself. I didn't just explore the causes of dysarthria on the net, I researched all the items on the list. Whilst there is no such thing as an acceptable terminal illness, this disease, this MND, makes even doctors shudder.

'Do me a favour Nig.'

'What?'

'When you go on the net to research MND, let's do it together.'

'OK.'

As Nigel steers the car towards the A64, I rehearse tomorrow's dialogue with the kids.

'Motor neurone disease?' they'll say. 'What's that?'

The kids, like Nigel, won't have heard of it. It's rare. But I had heard of it. And when Peter Harrop uttered those three dreadful words, the memory of a documentary I watched years ago charged into my mind and refused to leave. I had made a cuppa in anticipation of some senseless programme, something like *Who Wants to Be a Millionaire*, and I happened upon that week's *Panorama*, as I settled down to wait. Those images, as vivid as if they were being screened in front of me right now, captivate me once more.

...

She's such a tiny woman. Appears a bit odd. Kind of crooked.

My God, they're making a job and a half of lifting her out of that chair. Is she really so heavy? Two of them, struggling with her. Hope they're not hurting her, dragging her up like that. She's a dead weight. Incapable of helping. Unable to move. Must be like she's made of lead. Look at her, poor thing. There ought to be some kind of lifting equipment for people like this. Surely?

What's that awful noise? Is she speaking? Sounds like a trapped animal wailing in fright, I've never heard such a pitiful noise. The desperate woman must be brain damaged. Has to be. I'm amazed they can understand her at all. She must be in pain. Listen to her.

Oh, it's unwatchable. This is shocking. She's drooling. That must be her husband. How lovely, wiping the drool from her lips with such tenderness. He must love her so very much. This is heart breaking.

She must have had a stroke. Bound to. Ah, no, not a stroke. Motor neurone disease. Whatever that is. Yes, of course, the Stephen Hawking thing. Wonder how old she is? Fiftyish? She seems older. Exhausted. The poor buggers. She's begging to die. Campaigned for months for a doctor to help her but the courts won't allow it. Bastards. She longs to die with dignity, at home. Praying for this misery to stop. Hell, who could blame her? State she's in. I would. Unbearable. What must it be like to suffer like that? I can't begin to imagine. The entire family must be devastated. Poor wretches. Thank God this kind of thing happens to other people. Not people like us.

I recall the horror I felt at the dreadful roar she made as she tried to speak. It haunts me still. I remember the pity, as I witnessed those disturbing scenes of personal tragedy. Now, I am wracked with shame. Only happens to other people, I'd thought. Not people like us. Nothing like that could ever happen to us. Oh yes it could. It is. It's happening to us. To Nigel.

...

I glance towards Nigel as he drives. His handsome face, concentrating on the road. He grips the steering wheel with a lightness belying those strong, work-worn hands. His driving is smooth, swift and competent. How long before driving is beyond him? Until walking isn't an option? How long before his body is consumed, withered and destroyed by this disease? How long before Nigel's speech is displaced by a haunting, unintelligible clamour? And will he, like the pitiable woman in the programme, reach the point where his torment is so great he longs for death? Will he be allowed to make the choices denied her?

An hour ago, lunch was our primary concern. Could it be true that, now, this is our future? Yes, it could. So, how do we tell the kids?

7

BREAKING THE NEWS

Within an hour of telling Craig there were more tests to be done we could hardly show up at his home and say, 'Sorry, that's not the case.' I ignore two calls from Ellie. I imagine her fury and regret not answering her calls, but I can't pretend things are alright when they aren't. And, I'm not ready. I don't know what to say or how to say it. Just as Nigel, caught off guard, having had no time to process the dreadful news, responded to Craig's question without thinking. I guess Ellie, frustrated, phoned Craig and he inadvertently perpetuated the lie. In turn, she informed Becky and now, the grim news we must impart to the kids feels even more harrowing.

That night, Nigel and I consume sufficient alcohol around our kitchen table for us to expect at least a couple of hours of welcome oblivion. Yet, sleep abandons us. The endless night creeps by, each excruciating second drags like an hour; every hour, a lifetime. On our second cup of tea, we prop ourselves up against the pillows, gazing at our reflection in the mirrored wardrobes lining the wall before us. Expressionless eyes stare back at us from deep hollows in grey, deadpan faces. We could pass for a pair of apprentice ghouls at a 'how to improve your spookiness' convention.

At 3.00 a.m., I give up all hope of sleep and stand under a hot shower. I clean the bathroom, gather the washing and set a load going. In the kitchen, I empty the dishwasher before reloading it with the few mugs and side plates from our nocturnal tea and biscuits. I prowl through the house without purpose. No need for the customary haste in completing mundane tasks before dashing off to work. No rush. No work today. I wipe the already clean surfaces and switch the kettle on yet again. Coffee this time. And paracetamol.

Nigel is out of bed. He's huddled in the brown, buttoned leather office chair at the desk in the hallway, custom-made to accommodate the computer, printer and usual home study paraphernalia. We spend a lot of our time here in this practical, inviting space. Oak bookshelves store the compilations of hard-backed Reader's Digest novels, accumulated since we were first married. There are several 'how to' books and popular fiction located amongst an imposing collection of battered old volumes of *The War Illustrated*: a couple of which once substituted for the broken leg of our first bed. Nigel's golfing trophies, primarily clocks and glassware, are displayed between ornaments. On top of the shelves, a bust of Shakespeare dominates one end and Apollo, the other. In the centre is a cheerful sculpture of the three wise monkeys. On the wall behind the computer, providing moments of contemplation when your eyes stray from the screen, is a framed poem written by Nigel's mum, Dorreen, to mark her fiftieth birthday. There is a studious photograph of me holding two intellectual tomes and wearing a borrowed cap and gown, along with a scholastic mood-inspiring print of a magnificent old book-lined library, complete with librarian standing atop a pulpit ladder, engrossed in the book held before his face, whilst clutching another between his knees and a third tucked beneath his arm.

The blue-green light from the computer screen illuminates Nigel's face in the surrounding darkness. His hand cups the mouse as he manoeuvres the icon, hovering over the websites listed there, before a click denotes he has made his choice.

'Motor neurone disease. Neurological condition.'

Ah. He didn't wait, as I asked. No matter, I'm here now.

Without speaking, I place his coffee and paracetamol, should he need them, next to the mouse mat.

'Thanks,' he says, not diverting his eyes from the screen.

I stand behind him and rest my hand on his shoulder. For the next two hours the silence is punctured by the click-click of the mouse and the dull throbbing of the kitchen clock as it counts the seconds towards the dawn. I gaze at the screen as he researches one website after another, reads article after article on motor neurone disease and views every related video on YouTube.

We learn MND is a rare disorder, affecting around 5000 people in the UK at any one time. The cells which control movement, are gradually destroyed as the body is overwhelmed by a brutal, creeping paralysis. Nigel's muscles will deteriorate until he can't move, speak, swallow, eat, or breathe. We don't know the route it will take. There is no predictable pattern. Each individual is different. The websites talk of 'personal journeys' like you're setting off on some kind of adventure. Some people first lose the function in their legs, some their arms. Others lose the ability to speak and swallow. Some drop dead before their limbs are affected at all. It could kill you in six months or it could linger for years. More than fifty percent of people with MND die within fourteen months.

Nigel's lucky therefore. His prognosis of three to five years is the best you can expect. Whatever the timescale, whatever route the journey takes, there'll be nobody at the end asking if you had an enjoyable trip. No matter who you are, the outcome is the same: the inability to breathe, and ultimately, death.

MND strikes at random. No reason. No trigger. Man or woman, often, though not always, over fifty years old, in good physical shape and one who leads an active lifestyle. Nigel fits the profile. Professional athletes around the world succumb to the disease. Not a threat to your average couch potato, it would appear.

As we peruse the long and complex process of diagnosis, we recognise the gamut of tests Nigel endured. Like the doctor said, the tests are designed to eliminate other diseases. There is no single, conclusive test for MND. Well, that's not true. There is one: an autopsy.

'I bet Doctor Harrop knew what you had the second you walked into his office,' I whisper.

'Yes, he probably did.'

Nigel finds the BBC *Panorama* article, which has haunted me since his diagnosis, 'Please help me die.' Dianne Pretty's desperate plea. This helpless 43-year-old woman, who could communicate only by pressing a pad on a machine called a light writer, talks of a life worse than death. Incontinent, unable to move or hold a cup; unable to scratch an itch or control the saliva drooling from her mouth; her cry, when striving to speak, a grunt becoming a low-pitched scream that could be heard half-way down her street. Described in the article as 'a howl that made the hairs stand up at the back of your neck – like the sound of an animal being tortured.'

I close my eyes. Not sure I can endure any more. Nigel, converse-ly, is determined to face this and he reads on. Stephen Hawking, diagnosed in 1963 when just twenty-one. Still here forty-four years later. Does this offer hope? If you're content to be trapped within a depleted body and exist solely within the confines of your mind, then maybe.

Nigel comes across the documentary on YouTube of Craig Ewart, a man from Harrogate, suffering from MND, who, in September 2006, travelled with his wife Mary to Dignitas in Switzerland, to commit accompanied suicide. How appalling must this thing be for death to be so desired?

'Poor man,' I say.

'Not a bad way to go,' says Nigel.

As we share Craig Ewart's final moments and see him slip into eternal darkness, the first golden rays of dawn illuminate the hallway, alerting us to the birth of a new day. No matter what personal tragedy or unspeakable horror occurs, the sun never ceases to rise. I wish this absolute certainty, this new dawn, could fill me with hope that Nigel's journey won't be anything near as unbearable as some. Yet there's not a sliver of hope for us to cling to, in anything we've seen tonight.

With the dawn comes the strident, choking calls summoning the squabble of seagulls to the sea. The squealing chorus intensifies as the sky is filled with the squawks and hoots of excited gulls eager to follow the fishing fleet. Many ignore the call, and perch instead on rooftops and chimney pots. One of them alights on our garden wall and struts along its length, puffing out its chest and caw, caw, cawing – a shrieking siren – mocking the frenzied activity in the skies above him. This one will be among those gulls who prefer their fish already battered, and who will gorge on scraps of fried fish and chips snatched from unemptied litter bins, or, as is increasingly the case, straight from the hands of unguarded tourists.

The discordant racket outside is as disturbing and as unwelcome as the material contained in those MND articles.

'That's enough,' I say, planting a kiss on the top of Nigel's head.

He wavers for a second, the cursor hovering over the next video. 'OK, for now,' he says, closing the screen and standing up.

I reach for him and we embrace, holding each other close. I need his strong arms around me and take a moment to still the churning in my guts. When we part, I cup his face in my hands, 'Are you OK?' I ask, struggling to read his expression. What's going on inside his head? How is he processing all this?

Now, his gentle hands cup my face. The lenses of his glasses are smudged with fingerprints and the dark shadows beneath his tired eyes transform their usual bluish green to a steel grey. He kisses the tip of my nose and says, 'Julie, everybody gets a kick in the bollocks at some point. This is mine.'

I am not surprised by Nigel's pragmatic response to his situation. He manages the heartaches life throws at him with the same spirit as he welcomes the joys. I'm reminded of a line from Rudyard Kipling's 'If-':

If you can meet with triumph and disaster

And treat those two imposters just the same.

'Some kick,' I say.

'Yeah,' he acknowledges as he strokes my hair. 'It is.' He grips my shoulders and we stand, facing each other. 'I'm packing in work,' he says. 'I'll speak to Glyn this morning.'

This isn't your first kick in the bollocks, I think, as Nigel heads for the shower. His life was touched by tragedy when he was a mere twenty years old. A soldier serving with the Army, he and his young wife Linda and new-born son Craig were based in Belfast, against a backdrop of bombings and riots, during the Troubles of the early seventies. This tumultuous posting was coming to an end and the regiment scheduled for Germany. Perhaps it was the anxiety at the thought of separation from her husband, or perhaps it was post-natal depression: a condition so easily overlooked in those days. But one night, without warning, Linda took enough pills to kill her in her sleep. The inquest ruled the death 'misadventure.' Whatever demons may lurk within him, Nigel keeps them hidden. This episode in his life has remained private, and whilst never regarded as a secret, or concealed from the children, neither has it been discussed at length. Craig was a delightful, five month old baby when I first peered over the side of his cot and marvelled at his innocent, sleeping face. Falling in love with him required no effort at all.

I prepare breakfast. Scrambled eggs. I need something to beat.

...

Nigel is on the phone when I walk into the bedroom. 'It's motor neurone disease. Yeah. Motor neurone disease. No, there's no point. Anyway, we're off to the pub at teatime if you want to come. Yeah, OK. See you later.' He ends the call.

'Who was that?' I ask.

'Craig.'

'What did he say?'

'Not a lot. Asked if I'd any more doctor's appointments.'

I perch on the edge of the bed, 'You told him like that?'

'Like what?'

'Like you just did. "It's motor neurone disease," no explanation. Nothing.' I strive to conjure up Craig's thoughts during that phone call. Was he confused? Bewildered? Or the opposite: unconcerned? 'I thought we'd planned to tell Craig face-to-face.'

Nigel draws an exasperated breath and flops down beside me on the bed. 'Look, I phoned him and asked him to come for a cup of tea. He said he needed to finish a job before it rains. What could I do?'

'Alright, I'm sorry. I don't know. Had he heard of it? Did he understand what it means?'

Nigel clasps my hands within both of his. 'He didn't say. I doubt it. It's not possible to make things any better, is it?'

I gaze at the face of the man I love. Those eyes, normally alight with mischief, are clouded with worry.

'But Craig won't appreciate the seriousness of it. He'll have no idea.'

'Well he's coming here before we go to the pub, so we'll tell him then,' says Nigel, kissing my forehead before leaving the bedroom.

I remain seated on the bed a while longer, and consider how we've managed to mess up the first step of telling the kids. I don't blame Nigel – it's not his fault. A mere twenty-four hours since we learned Nigel has MND, I suppose he's unable to process it himself, never mind explain it to anybody else.

I imagine Craig puzzling over the nature of the disease. It will nag at him. Between cleaning windows, he might ring Charlotte, and ask her if she's heard of it. Get her to look on the net. If it rains, as expected, he might pop home and do it himself. And he'll know.

Two hours later, Craig walks through the door. One glance at his handsome face, so like his dad's, tells me that's exactly what he did.

'I had no idea it was that bad,' he says, as I fold him into my arms.

...

The Indigo Alley boasts 'live ale and real music'. The exterior is unremarkable: a doorway leading from the pavement, easily over-looked but for the bright indigo paintwork. At the end of North Marine Road, opposite the fire station, and within easy staggering distance of a choice of Chinese and Indian restaurants. This is our 'go to' pub, or, to be more accurate, the only pub we go to, and the publicans, Graham and Irene, are friends.

Inside, it claims to be nothing other than a pub. A large, open plan room, with a practical, bare wooden floor. The space is sepa-rated into left and right by the central front door and the passage to the toilets. The area to the left is is reserved predominantly for regular, live bands. The bar, all wood and glass, fills the back wall on the right side of the room. A few bar stools are scattered beneath the far window, but this is a pub where drinkers are expected to stand. Apart from the occasional tray of sandwiches and pork pies, brought out to keep people drinking when there's a major rugby match on, no food is served here.

I glance at the clock behind the bar. 4.30 p.m. Still too early to ring the girls. They won't be home from work.

Apart from a couple of regulars, the place is ours. Despite not being a drinker, Craig elected to join us. Now he shadows Nigel like a bodyguard, unable to leave his side. The protective instinct appears triggered in Paula also, as her anxious gaze flits between Nigel and me, as though preparing to catch us should one of us col-lapse. Every few minutes, she releases her hand from her husband Tom's grasp, to pat and stroke my back. Les, who, under normal circumstances would be regaling the gathering with his personal interpretation of the day's news, the state of the country or the incompetence of the government, stands, along with his partner Sally, in shocked silence. The news has aged him, aggravating the sharpness of his features. Deep furrows etch into pointed cheekbones and sunken eyes stare from a sallow face.

The snippets of exchanges I overhear include, 'It's unbelievable.' 'How could this happen?' 'It can't be true.' 'What the fuck is MND anyway?' And 'Poor Nig.'

Glyn leans on the bar, his face crunched in a severe scowl. Graham is drying pint glasses with a cloth. He keeps shaking his head. Bruce, a regular, occupies the corner spot, and as Nigel leans on the bar ordering another round of drinks, I overhear, 'So what is it mate? A stroke?' No need to catch Nigel's answer to register the shock on Bruce's face, and I don't need to be a lip reader to recognise the words, 'Oh no. Fucking hell, I'm so sorry mate.' Graham rejects the money Nigel proffers for the drinks. He knows.

It's time. I slip away from my group and head for the toilet. It's freezing in here. I must ask Irene to install a radiator, or at least a towel rail. Anything to take the edge off the chill. There are two cubicles, both empty. Shivering, I lock myself in one of them and plonk down on the toilet seat. Not a desirable setting for the news I'm about to impart.

Ellie answers her phone on the second ring. Her anxiety and hint of irritation is evident in her expectant 'Hello?'

'Hi, it's me.'

'Yes.'

'Sorry for not answering your calls yesterday.'

'OK.'

'Your dad doesn't need any more tests.'

'What? But Craig said – '

'I know, we didn't intend to mislead Craig, it just came out.'

'Well, what then?' says Ellie, the irritation dissipated.

There's no other way than to say it. 'It's motor neurone disease.'

'What's that?'

I knew it. 'Erm, it's complicated,' I say, conscious I'm not handling this well. I still don't know how to describe it.

'What do you mean complicated?' she says. 'Boys! Stop it!'

I hear Ben and Tom, scrapping in the background. 'It's to do with nerves and muscles. The muscles become weak over time. There's no cure. It's not good.'

'No cure? Will Dad be OK?'

A second's pause. 'No.'

'Oh, no,' she says, her voice breaking. 'How's Dad?'

'He's fine. Incredible. You know your dad. I'm so sorry we're not with you right now.'

'Boys! For God's sake!'

'Listen, darling. Might be best if you look on the net. It's all there.' I struggle to recall a specific website, as there's nothing good in any of them. 'Google it, and we'll talk tomorrow.' We end the call as someone comes into the toilet. I'm not ringing Becky here, I'll go outside when I've swallowed more liquid courage. And it's warmer in the street than in the loos.

'Becky, it's Mum, how are you?'

'Oh, I'm alright,' she groans. 'I've not had a bloody minute. I've been back from Malawi for two days and they've shoved me in this dog-shit room. I've a load of bags to unpack and there's crap all over the place.'

Oh dear. This is awful. She's already close to tears and I've barely started.

'Don't suppose you've spoken to Ellie, or Craig?'

'No, haven't had chance. Why?'

'It's your dad.'

'Oh yeah, course, sorry, how is he? What did the doctor say?'

And, as with Ellie, there's no other way than to say it. 'It's motor neurone disease.'

'What's that?'

The rest of the conversation goes the same as with Ellie, except Becky is unable to choke back the tears.

'I don't want Dad to be poorly,' she says, becoming a little girl again.

'I know darling,' I say, before suggesting, as I did with Ellie, that she Google motor neurone disease.

'No. No way.'

'Really?' I thought the younger generation Googled every blessed thing. 'OK, maybe you could ring Ellie and Craig. Could you visit Ellie this weekend?'

'No. I can't. I don't know. I'll see.'

My heart breaks for Becky. She's all alone. Craig's and Ellie's families can provide support and distraction, whilst Becky has nobody at all there for her now. She'll go to bed for the weekend. That's what she does when she's upset: sleeps at it.

I head back into the warmth of the pub. Well, that went well.

Shit, shit, shit, fucking shit!

The alcohol flows steadily for the remainder of the evening and proves to be an effective anaesthetic as, once we've staggered home, Nigel is in bed and asleep before I'm undressed. I'm not ready for sleep. I idle in the kitchen in my pyjamas and gaze at the collages I made from Ellie's and Danny's wedding photographs in 1998 and Craig's and Charlotte's in 2000. The collages tell the story from hen do to night do, and capture all the joyous celebrations in between. Ellie's and Danny's was such an elaborate, military affair, complete with guard of honour. Danny and the soldiers looked spectacular in their ceremonial Number Ones. Navy with red stripes down the legs, red waistcoat and red band on the dress caps. To continue the theme, the bridesmaids wore stunning red gowns, navy suits for Nigel and me, red tie for Nigel and a vast flying saucer of a red hat for me. And there, in the centre of the collage, the embodiment of a princess straight out of a fairy tale, our delightful, incomparable daughter, the bewitching bride. Her lavish gown, with embroidered train and bardot neckline, enhancing her soft shoulders, captivated and reduced me to tears the second she tried it on. Shimmering, brunette ringlets are tucked behind the golden tiara she adored. Eleanor looked divine.

I close my eyes and relish the waves of memories as they flood over me. The interminable shopping trips, the months of planning around this table, the chaos on the morning of the wedding, the panic when the flowers arrived late, Nigel's three attempts to tie the perfect Windsor knot, his joy at the vision of his stunning daughter, the way he settled her nerves and made her giggle, his pride, profound and well deserved, as he led her down the aisle.

In the bottom right-hand corner of the collage, there is the picture of a tearful Ellie, standing before the red Transit van, which would take her away from us, and drive her and her new husband to Fallingbostel in Germany, where Danny would take up his posting.

'I'm so glad they're home, now,' I whisper.

Two years later, it's Craig's special occasion. Craig, so like Nigel, with his dark, cropped hair, striking blue eyes framed with abundant lashes and heavy brows, also shares his dad's humour and ready wit. Socially adept and bursting with confidence, Craig was tongue-tied and self-conscious when called upon to make his speech. Of similar build, although a tad taller than his dad – thanks to the straight legs – and as strong, as a result of carrying and climbing ladders. Craig and his lovely wife Charlotte, slim and so petite, her crimson and gold bouquet of trumpet lilies almost as tall as her, beam with happiness as they pose for the camera, her brown hair curled behind Ellie's tiara. Photographs of the many guests radiate from the centre. The men in the family, all of whom opted to wear suits of varying shades of blue, adopt the classic male, wide-legged stance, reminiscent of bouncers, with hands clasped protectively before their bits.

Two marvellous, magical days. Now, nine years on we are grand-parents to Ellie's boys, Ben and Tom, and Craig's girls, Jemma and Amy. I pore over these treasured collages, reliving those jubilant moments, and as I stare at the images, my delight shrivels like dry, smouldering leaves, into despair.

Will Nigel live to see Becky marry? Will she find love in time for him to share her special day? Will he, for a third time, experience the joy of knowing his precious child is happy? All we have learned today, tumbles, like troops of stampeding acrobats, unbidden into my mind. Besieged, I close my eyes against the torrent and rest my frazzled head in my hands. How long have we got? How long has Nigel left to live?

Tonight, the comforting warmth of our battered old pine table serves as my pillow. And once again, the cracks are filled with tears.

8

HAVE I TOLD YOU THE ONE ABOUT THE POLAR BEAR?

Death has moved in. It oozes through doors, leaks through the letterbox, bleeds through brickwork, weeps through windows. It skulks in the corners of every room. It drips from ceilings and clings to carpets. It prowls in passages and shivers in shadows. It lurks in cupboards, the fridge and the pantry. It swirls in my coffee in the morning and I taste it as I drain my glass of wine at night. Like a putrid smell, it permeates our home and, like poison, it contaminates all it touches.

This intruder, this unwelcome alien, has taken a seat at our table, declared its intentions, and settled down to wait. Nothing any of us can say or do will make it leave. It besieges Nigel. Consumes him. Its presence so profound that when I look at Nigel that's all I see. I percieve its reflection in the haunted, frightened eyes of my family. We stare at Nigel, all of us, eager to retain the image of him whilst he's strong. Handsome. Upright. We need to lock that image deep in our memories. Before he disappears.

The news, as they say, is out. It ripped through the family with the destructive force of a tornado. Now, we are struggling through the wreckage the best we can.

Craig devotes all his spare time to his dad. He can't leave him alone for long. Ellie, following my phone call, plunged head-first into the web and emerged, hours later, devastated. Becky still spurns the net. Neither will she discuss it. She's not ready to know. Both girls arrange leave and are on their way home.

Les calls in daily. He slumps at the kitchen table, bewildered.

'Are they sure?' he asks. 'Could it be a mistake?'

Mel, unable to speak when Nigel gave her the news over the phone, had to find the words to inform Tracey, at her home in Tenerife, and their poor dad, Ron, holidaying there. Their distance makes this beyond unbearable.

'Thank God Mum isn't still with us,' they say. 'She couldn't cope with this.'

I'm not so sure. Dorreen – a woman typical of her time – strong, forthright and practical, would conceal her own heartache and support Nigel and her family through this nightmare. The kids didn't call her 'Super Doz' for nothing.

When Paula wakes in the mornings, she is inexplicably surrounded by 'Quality Street' wrappers. She has no recollection of raiding the goody jar in the middle of the night. Mum's pristine home is left to gather dust whilst she also uncharacteristically devours chocolate. My dad, who likes to believe the world is kind and just, is struggling to accept it. It's not supposed to be like this.

Family and friends phone to offer us comfort and support and afterwards phone each other, in the hope of finding some for themselves. The news weighs like a boulder in the pit of our bellies. It's heavy, cumbersome, and impossible to comprehend. Why Nigel?

How did this happen? If I understand, perhaps I'll handle it better. There must be a reason. There has to be. Like despairing, starving wretches, we gorge on every scrap there is to be found on the internet. They should tell you which websites to research when faced with such a diagnosis. The majority of sites are terrifying. One of the best, the 'Motor Neurone Disease Association', guides you through the labyrinth in a protective, tactful way. It talks of living with MND, not dying from it. The site warns you not to click on a particular link if you'd prefer not to know the prognosis. Inspiring stories of the achievements of fellow sufferers are championed on its platform. It offers practical support, guidance and encouragement. But it doesn't offer hope.

Despite not wishing to be members of this particular club, we've joined the association. After all, when you are lost and somebody hands you a map, you take it. They've sent us a file. A bright blue, A4, lever arch file, resembling, to my dismay, a welcome pack. It screams: organise yourselves. There's a section for listing the contact details of the myriad of medical professionals who will forthwith form part of our lives, a section explaining all the equipment Nigel will ultimately need, stuff we didn't know existed, all designed to compensate for a failing body. A section on overcoming the challenges in communication, one focusing on the difficulties of eating and drinking, and finally, end of life decisions. That section is missing. Mistake or deliberate, I wonder?

It reminds me of the portfolios our students compile for their national vocational qualifications. Nigel reads through it before pushing it aside. I banish the file in the cupboard beneath the computer for now. We're not ready for that world yet. Maybe later. Much, much later.

For all that, the world we're not ready to be part of is knocking at our door. A nurse from the palliative care team at Scarborough's St Catherine's Hospice pays us a visit. Vanessa is in her mid-thirties, short, light-brown crop and heavy rimmed glasses. She explains this is her sole visit as she's leaving palliative care to train as a vicar. Nigel manages a polite, 'Oh, fascinating,' grunt, and asks where she will study. There's a theological college in Durham, she explains, her hometown. Saves Nigel the bother of asking her where she's from. I ponder the Mrs Vicar role and wonder if she has a Mister. Will he arrange the flowers in the church, bake the cakes and man the bric-a-brac stall at the village fete? Or, what if the Mister is a Mrs? Now, that'll set the tongues a-wagging.

'I'm here to set up your file, so you're on the system,' says Vanessa. This MND demands a lot of admin.

'Don't fancy being part of that system,' says Nigel.

'No, I understand,' she says, before adding, 'Would you like to come and look round the hospice?'

Er, no. Not ready for that either.

'You'd be surprised. It's a happy place,' she insists, regarding our blank faces.

In fact, all her language is positive. Subtle, yet something taught as standard, I assume, as I do. Like the MNDA website, she refers to living with MND, not suffering or dying from it. She talks of the kind of support the hospice will provide as his illness progresses, not worsens. And when Nigel becomes less well, as opposed to more ill.

'I want to die at home,' says Nigel, calmly sipping his tea. He could be remarking on the weather.

'Of course,' she says, scribbling in her book. 'We will help you with that.'

Are all our conversations going to be this weird from now on?

'Nice woman considering she's a God-botherer,' says Nigel, when Vanessa leaves us.

'I suppose "nice" is a necessity in that job, Nig. I can't imagine being a vicar.'

'Not believing in God might prove a problem,' he says.

'True.'

I'm not sure I'm up to this. I've had a life free of tragedy. I'm terrified. I'm unable to utter the words 'motor neu...' without tears clogging my throat. Performing anything other than basic functions is out of the question and I've taken time off work.

Each morning is like waking from an anaesthetic. I'm numb, confused. Familiar things appear unfamiliar. My muddled mind searches for memories of yesterday, something to clarify today. Death, having stolen the space in the bed between Nigel and me, says, 'Good morning. Did you imagine I was but a dream?' And it all comes hurtling back.

There are days when Nigel is so restless I fear his pacing will wear a groove in the kitchen floor. I imagine he's dodging the monsters inside his head. If he keeps moving, he'll hold them off. If he stands still, they'll overpower him, and he'll be lost. Apart from not working, he's carrying on as usual. He plays golf, rides his bike, calls at the pub. Today, Nigel and Craig are at the Indigo watching the rugby. Craig is no fan of rugby and no fan of the pub either, however the need to be with his dad supersedes what he dislikes. Perhaps if they do normal blokey things they'll share father and son time and drive away the killer.

Alone, I hide behind the settee. Squeeze into the tiniest space. Room only for me. Nothing will hurt me here. Nothing will find me. Just as monsters can't find you beneath the duvet, I'm safe. Our new adversary, Death, wouldn't think to look for me here.

The doorbell rings. I ignore it. Ellie and Becky are not due for another two hours. I've locked the doors. I can't face anybody. I need to crouch here, behind the settee, and press my face into the carpet. I need the strange and woeful noises smothered deep within me to erupt at last. My throat won't hold them captive any longer. I can't swallow any more sobs. I crave this time, this hour, to let it all out. I need to wail.

A lot of wailing has taken place these last few weeks, amongst us women that is. Not akin to Jews at the Wall, or the howling display of grief common in Islamic and Arabic cultures, or the keening of the Irish and Scottish, more a typical, English expression of sorrow, released following the consumption of unlimited quantities of alcohol.

Later, I open the door to Ellie and Becky. There they stand, arm in arm at the foot of the steps, peering at me with anguished, tear-filled eyes. They appear younger, childlike.

'Mum,' quakes Ellie, in a tight, hesitant voice. She attempts a smile, bites hard on her bottom lip.

I open my arms wide. Becky's face crumples and both girls, unable to contain their sobs, rush into my embrace. I stroke their hair, squeeze their shoulders and kiss their tear-stained cheeks and whisper, 'It will be okay.' We hold each other until they manage to control their snuffles. Ellie first.

'How's Dad?' she says, her sea green eyes still glistening with tears.

'He's amazing. So brave. As you'd expect of your dad.'

'And Craig?' she says, 'I've spoken to him on the phone, he sounded in a bit of a state.'

'I know, he's struggling to deal with it. Your dad is his hero, after all.'

'He's part of the reason I came home to be honest,' adds Ellie.

'Bless you, darling,' I say, tucking an escaped strand of coffee-coloured hair behind her ear. 'He'll be grateful.' Ellie has inherited her dad's quiet strength. Very little fazes her. This is the young woman who thought nothing of driving across Europe from Germany to Scarborough when Danny served in Iraq for four months, two babies in the car, no mobile phone, no sat nav, just a creased up old road map. As one who shudders at the prospect of driving as far as London, I marvel at her.

'What's going to happen?' whispers Becky, all five feet nothing of her, the personification of a cute Action Girl doll in her combat uniform and black boots. I glimpse the white mesh laundry bag slung over her shoulder and stroke her cheek with my thumb as I take it from her. No matter how difficult things are, the laundry must be done. Her long, mahogany tinted hair is corralled in a tidy bun at the nape of her neck, the beret somehow stays in place on her petite head and her fearful eyes, brown, like mine, search for answers.

'I don't know. It's impossible to know for sure.' I place my arms around their shoulders and guide them into the kitchen. 'Come on, Dad and Craig will be back soon.'

When Nigel arrives home, he hugs his daughters while they fight to hold back fresh tears.

'It's lovely to see you,' he says. 'But you needn't have made a special trip.'

It is possibly the most stupid thing I've ever heard him say. Craig cradles his sisters and, as is so often the case, we gather round the kitchen table. Nigel has a beer, Ellie, Becky and me, pinot grigio, and a pint of tonic water for Craig.

'I've got three to five,' Nigel says. 'I apologise now if I'm a nasty bastard at any point along the way.'

'You've always been a nasty bastard,' laughs Craig.

'Don't be daft,' says Ellie. 'No need to apologise for anything.

'You're allowed to be as nasty as you like,' says Becky.

'Well,' he continues, 'If things get too bad, there's always Dignitas.'

We fall silent and peer at him, unspoken questions on our lips. He laughs and dismisses his words with a flick of his hand. We disregard the Dignitas comment. He's joking, as always.

'Anyway, I've started a bucket list. Top of the list: an earring.'

'An earring?' echo the girls.

'A bloody earring? You?' says Craig.

'Finally,' I say. 'Your macho dad's wanted one forever. Fancies himself as a bit of a pirate.'

'For God's sake, don't choose one of those bloody diamante things,' says Craig. 'You'll look a right wanker.'

'No, I won't, I'm thinking a hoop.'

'Make sure they shove it in the left ear, not the right,' advises Ellie.

'Why?' I ask. 'What's it matter?'

'Only gays wear earrings in their right ear.'

Nigel and I exchange 'well fancy that' glances.

'I'll come with you to Claire's Accessories tomorrow and sort it,' says Becky.

'Is that it?' asks Craig. 'An earring. Nowt else?'

'No. Number two on the list: a Jag.'

'Well that's more like it. I'll come with you to choose that,' says Craig, clinking his glass of tonic water against Nigel's beer.

'OK, we'll drive to York tomorrow. The nearest dealer is at Clifton Moor.'

'After the earring,' interjects Becky.

'Bloody hell,' says Craig, 'deal with the important stuff first, eh?'

'What's number three?' asks Ellie.

Nigel takes a swig of his beer before answering. 'I want to play poker in Vegas.'

'Wow, fantastic,' says Becky, the one responsible for teaching him poker – specifically Texas Hold'em – on her return from a posting in Afghanistan, where, when not dodging mortars, she could be found at the poker table. The rest of us affirm our approval. If Nigel said he wanted a trip into space we'd find a way to make it happen.

'You'll come with me for that?' he asks, directing the question at me.

'Of course.'

'We'll travel business class and stay at the Wynn. It's a dead posh hotel, not like that shitty Bellagio.' Nigel had spent a long weekend at Las Vegas with a group of business associates a couple of years before.

'Then I'll definitely come with you. Is the Bellagio that shit?'

'It is compared to the Wynn.'

'Right, we'd better save up for a week of poker losses.'

'Or wins,' he says. 'But maybe not, you're probably right.'

'Is that it?' asks Becky, pouring herself another glass. 'Ellie?'

'Yes, thanks,' says Ellie holding her glass aloft and adding to Becky's question, 'Didn't you always want to visit Vietnam, Dad?'

Nigel leans back in the pine armchair and sips his beer.

'Yes, I'd love to see the Chu Chi tunnels.'

'What are they?' says Craig.

'A network of tunnels the Vietnamese utilised during the Vietnam War. Could be the reason it carried on so long. They're supposed to be fabulous.'

'So?' says Becky. 'Are you going?'

'I don't know, now,' Nigel says. 'I'm not sure I can stand spending a lot of time in airports, cramming in as many different countries as possible, before I die.'

This reference to his death halts the discussion and the three of them stare at their drinks.

'Sorry,' he says.

'Well, you've made a start,' I gush. 'It's not too shabby a list. And, here, the lasagne's ready.' I take the lasagne from the oven and place it in the centre of the table. It gives us something to do.

The rest of the evening passes like so many before. The beer and wine flow freely, as does the merriment. Precious family memories are recalled and retold, no doubt embellished, but definitely funnier than the original version. Craig entertains us with his outraged account of the occasion, when scaffolding with his dad, he misjudged the catch of a mere 21' pole.

'Bloody near ripped my hand off,' he says.

'Nah,' says Nigel. 'It was a scratch. And anyway, you should've caught it.'

'I was fourteen!'

'OK, fair enough.'

'And,' laughs Craig, 'when you finally took me to hospital, at the end of the bloody day, you said to tell 'em I fell off my bike.'

Ellie shares with us her earliest memories of Nigel singing her still favourite song, *As Tears Go By*, in the bath, as he washed away the smell of muck, fags and beer. Without fail, he would call for her to fetch the sugar and washing up liquid to scrub the ingrained oil from his blackened palms.

'Why didn't you keep sugar and washing up liquid in the bathroom, Mum?' she says.

'I've no idea. It never occurred to me.' Nor can I understand why I didn't buy some Swarfega, a product which would doubtless do the job better, and save on sugar and washing up liquid. As it was, we didn't have a lot of money, and as my dad would say, 'necessity is the mother of invention.'

'Why didn't you just take them with you Dad?' she says.

'Who would listen to my singing if I did that?'

Becky remembers the time he drove to Lincoln after she'd phoned home in tears.

'I was convinced I couldn't hack the RAF. You took me out for a drink and stayed in my barrack room all night. You've always been a soft arse.'

Smiling at the memories, I pass Nigel another beer and fill our glasses with wine. Craig declines more tonic water.

'Anyway, have I told you the one about the polar bear?' says Nigel.

'A million times,' I say.

'Not the polar bear joke,' groans Craig. 'You've told that joke all my life.'

'I've never heard it,' says Becky.

'What?' says Ellie. 'You must have.'

'No I haven't,' she insists.

Here we go. Nigel takes a deep breath and prepares himself for the telling of his favourite joke. The older and cornier a joke is, the more he loves it. The 'what's brown and sticky? A stick,' has him in bits. He's already chuckling with mirth and anticipation as he collects his thoughts. I doubt he'll make it to the punch line. He rarely does. The telling of the joke is always more entertaining than the joke itself.

'There's this baby polar bear ...'

'Yeah.'

'And he says to his dad, "Dad, am I a real polar bear?"'

'Yeah.'

'And his dad says, "Of course you are son." And the baby polar bear says, "No, I mean a real polar bear, a proper, genuine, pukka polar bear."'

That's as far as he gets before his shoulders tremble and his face burns purple as he tries to control the convulsions. It's hopeless. He can't suppress the giggles. He throws his head back, abandoning himself to the joy of the moment and howls with laughter. Craig buries his head in his hands in mock exasperation and bangs his forehead on the table. His own jokes are equally appalling although he succeeds in reaching the end without the hysterics. Ellie chuckles along with her dad and Becky remains transfixed.

'Go on, Nige,' I say. 'You can do it.'

Nigel drags himself up in the chair, takes a swig of beer, "Of course you are, son,"' he squeaks between chortles. "' Why do you ask?"'

'Wait for it,' says Craig, without lifting his head.

'And the baby polar bear says, "I'm ..."'

'Oh, he's not gonna make it,' says Ellie as Nigel collapses in a crumpled heap, spilling some of his beer on Craig's head.

'Bollocks,' Craig says, jumping up, deftly catching the tea towel I chuck in his direction.

Nigel rubs his eyes and stutters an apology. 'Sorry.' He tries again. '"I'm ..."'

'Not happening,' says Ellie.

'This had better be good,' says Becky.

Craig dries the beer from his head. 'It isn't.'

'Come on Nige,' I say, willing him to make it to the end.

He takes a mighty breath and summons all his self-control to deliver the punch line, his voice a desperate, high-pitched squeal,

'"I'm fucking freezing!"'

'Oh God,' snorts Craig.

'Yey,' I applaud. 'Well done!'

'Never thought you'd finish,' says Ellie.

'Er, oh yes, I have heard it,' says Becky, ducking out of the way of the soggy cloth flying at her head.

Later that evening, Craig collects the keyboard he keeps in his van for rehearsing new tunes on the days when rain prevents him from working, and we belt out Pink Floyd songs deep into the night. We discuss anything except MND. We enjoy each other's company and snub the unwelcome intruder. It will not spoil our special time. Yet, Craig still leaves with someone's black mascara smeared all over his white T-shirt.

In the main, we are strong. Like Nigel. The extent of his strength surprises even me. Not a single tear has he shed. Not one outburst of anger, not one indulgent second of self-pity. No 'why me,' 'poor me', 'life's not fair.'

He is preparing to face the future the only way he knows how. Head on. I believe he is facing it with courage, and heroic resolve. He disagrees. He says he's not in the least bit brave. He simply has no choice.

In contrast, I take tentative steps into this unfamiliar territory. Like walking on quicksand, each faltering footfall is perilous. It is Nigel who guides me, and the rest of us, through these wretched early days. He is the one holding us in his arms as we weep. He is the one who still makes us chuckle as he cracks atrocious jokes when each family member visits for the first time after hearing the news.

'I've been *dying* to see you,' he quips, when my brothers come.

We laugh, in spite of ourselves, and our spirits are lifted ever so slightly.

After thirty-two years of loving this man I am falling in love with him all over again. The journey he is embarking upon promises to present him with unimaginable challenges. Along the way he will lose the ability to do all the things he loves to do. The path he will follow may plunge him to depths of despair that will test his unconquerable spirit. The road may lead to intolerable torment and unspeakable suffering.

But wherever this journey takes him, I will be by his side.

9

SPAIN

Late February 2007

We need warmth. Sunshine. We need to escape the gloom. Not merely the intrinsic gloom of the February weather, more the saturating melancholy that drenches us. We're tired, drained. Consumed by thoughts of MND and sick of talking about it, we are worn out and weary of worrying. We need to flee. We need Spain.

This particular stretch of Andalucía's Costa del Sol is new to us. In the past, Marbella has been our magnet, but Nigel gambled with something new and booked us into the Atalaya Park Hotel, nestled between San Pedro de Alcantara and Estepona, chosen with the kind of research similar to sticking a pin on a map. His gamble has paid off. The area is easily as seductive as Marbella. We amble along San Pedro's promenade, pausing to sample the tempting cocktails or jugs of sangria from the chiringuitos along the route. We linger over lunch in the delightful mountain village of Benahavis and amble through the spell-binding, historic and narrow streets of Estepona. Strolling hand in hand, the sun on our backs, heading for nowhere in particular. Despite staying within easy distance of three stunning golf courses, we don't make the effort to play, nor do we bother with any nightlife. Instead, we absorb the soothing rays of the sun into our sallow skin and revel in its comforting, healing warmth.

As we leave behind Estepona's port and marina and scurry away from the pungent fish market, we come across a deserted cove.

'Let's head down there,' says Nigel.

To reach it we need to climb over a wall two-feet high on this side, dropping around four feet onto a significant expanse of rock armour.

'Are you kidding?' I say, glancing at the rocky defences and my flip flops.

'Yes, come on, let's do it.'

The simple presence of the armour explains why the cove is deserted and, I'm guessing, clambering over jagged rocks in flip-flops is no easy feat. All the same, Nigel bounds the wall in a single leap and stretches out his arm to guide me over, a huge grin lighting up his face. Rising to the challenge I grab his hand, plonk my bum on the wall and swing my legs over the other side and, as I do, a flip flop flies from my foot and disappears between the rocks.

'Ooops.' I cry, 'Shit.'

'I'll carry you,' says Nigel, determined to reach that cove even with me clinging to his back.

I reach down and retrieve my remaining flip flop and fling it across the armour where it also disappears. 'There. A flip is useless without its flop. Come on.'

For the first time in weeks, we feel alive. Giggling like kids, we brave that bridge of boulders. After an abundance of girlish squealing and 'Come on, you can do it' encouragement, we emerge at the other side like conquering heroes. We are giddy. Carefree. Having fun.

The enchanting cove wraps us within its rugged arms. The virgin sand stretches before us like a sheet of glistening glass. The sea, iridescent and inviting as an old friend, beckons. Crystal-clear waters cool and caress our bare feet as we paddle along the secluded shore. Nigel happens upon a half-buried stick and the irresistible urge to leave a mark prompts him to scratch his name into the wet surface. Next, he engraves my name alongside it and envelops both within the shape of a heart.

'Love you,' he whispers, smiling.

'Love you too.'

I embrace him and for a moment we stand in silence, cocooned and at ease in this magical place. Hidden from the rest of the world, safe in this secret bay, Nigel drops his guard.

'I always knew I'd never get old,' he whispers into my neck.

His shoulders shudder and he gasps. An involuntary sob escapes from somewhere deep inside him. He presses his face into my neck and holds me close and as one, we sink to our knees, in the sand. For the first time since his diagnosis, Nigel allows himself to weep. I hold him, as he grieves his loss, and contemplates the future he will never know. Our plans to share our old age are denied us. Our family, our children, somehow expected to carry on without him.

'Whatever is coming, we'll face it together,' I say.

'I know,' he says.

Silent, bar the swish of the sea, soothing in its timelessness, we kneel, huddled in each other's arms. As we hold each other, we sweep away the fearful images of the all-consuming sorrow, which may blight our future, and instead, focus on the certainty of right now.

'Let's not dwell on tomorrow,' says Nigel. 'Let's enjoy what we have.'

Whatever we will face, we will deal with it. For now, all that matters, is now. The future must wait.

10
THE BUCKET LIST

June 2007 – Las Vegas

Nigel takes his place at the large oval poker table and acknowledges his fellow players with a smile. Six men, four women, focused on one thing: winning. An ostensibly amiable, yet hardly classy bunch of various colour, shape, size and sophistication. At least nobody is gracing the table in a bathrobe tonight. Gone are the days when gents frequented casinos dressed in dinner jackets and ladies were sure to be bedecked in elegant and exclusive gowns. Shame. At least the dealer, clad in the black and gold casino livery, looks the part.

He swishes the new deck of cards in a perfect arc before placing them in the automatic shuffler. The woman to the left of Nigel, all baubles, brass and boobs, fiddles with her towers of chips. Perhaps she's down to the last of the housekeeping. Flanking Nigel's other side is a skinny guy wearing a cowboy hat, striped shirt and dazzling checked shorts. No fashionista here. His aggressive gum chewing brings to mind the snarling of a rabid dog. That would irritate the hell out of me but Nigel doesn't appear the least bit perturbed. He's loving this. With a spoonful of skill and a bucket load of luck he'll be here all night.

I spy on him from my vantage point at the doorway of the exclusive poker lounge. He appears at ease, chatting with the others, who seem to understand him. His slurred speech doubtless resonates, to the American ear, like a tipsy Prince Charles. He twirls the shiny new golden hoop in his left lobe. Still growing accustomed to it. He catches sight of me, and that practised poker face he adopts when gambling, erupts into a broad grin and he waves. I point at the ceiling signalling I'm going up to the room, make the thumbs up gesture for luck, blow him a kiss and leave him to it.

As I stroll along the plush and velvety highways of the small town which is our hotel, I elect to call for a nightcap at one of the dozen elaborate bars, sprinkled like glittering jewels along the seams of this lavish canvas. Nothing other than the remains of the book that didn't melt in the forty-two-degree heat by the pool, await me in the room. Might as well people watch for a while.

Skirting the punters playing blackjack at the bar, I find a quiet corner and take a moment to admire the artificial talons enhancing my now gorgeous hands. Do they warrant the hundred and forty dollars I forked out for them? Of course they don't. They'll be chewed off by Friday. And as for the ninety-dollar face cream resting in my bag, which swears to halt all further signs of ageing with a single application, well, I reckon I've been mugged.

Still, that is their business, after all. The town exists merely to relieve you of your money. However, it is done with such panache. Vegas is just as I expected: shameless in its hedonistic pursuits; decadent; stylish and garish.

We have sampled all Vegas has to offer. Sauntered along the Strip, dipping into a few of the sumptuous hotels to escape the oppressive heat. We journeyed to Egypt by way of the Luxor before popping over to Venice at the Venetian, where we declined a gondola ride in favour of a gelato. We side-stepped Celine Dion's performance at Caesar's Palace, choosing instead Monty Python's irreverent musical comedy, *Spamalot*. We were left underwhelmed by the sinking of the pirate ship at Treasure Island, but marvelled at the spectacular fountains of the Bellagio. However, Nigel is right, the Wynn has the edge. We revelled in the delectable tasting menu at the Wynn's 'Wing Lei' restaurant, where even my non-designer handbag was honoured with its own chair. Our fellow diners included Wayne Rooney and Colleen, neither of whom I recognised.

'He'll be here for the Ricky Hatton and Jose Luis Castillo fight,' said Nigel with such authority you could assume he had personally sold Mr Rooney his ticket.

We abandoned the hotels for the unmissable and thrilling, or terrifying if you're me, helicopter flight to the Grand Canyon and Hoover Dam. All in all, once you've exhausted the Strip and the shows, unless gambling is your thing, the fascination and the flamboyance of Vegas fades.

I set off to take a final peek at Nigel in the poker lounge. A lounge impossible to reach without the assault of the discordant din radiating from the gigantic lobby that is home to thousands of slot machines and aptly named one-armed bandits. These hotels may be palatial, but their lobbies, for me, are no more appealing than Scarborough's tacky amusement arcades. Unlike the hordes of witless worshippers, I am not tempted to slot a single cent into any one of these grotesque, guzzling gods. It takes a full ten minutes to flee from the chaotic cacophony and reach the relative tranquillity of the area reserved for more discerning gamblers.

Ah, pretty decent Nig, an impressive collection of chips. Increased his original stake by a considerable amount it would seem. He could well be here all night. He will stay for as long as it takes to lose all his chips. No doubt he will emerge at dawn, poorer in wealth, richer in joy.

It's been a super week. Earring sorted. Vegas sorted. Two out of three ticked off the bucket list.

...

August 2007 – Venice

Not on the list, but who doesn't want to see Venice?

Venice's San Clemente Palace swelters in the searing heat of the August sun. The hotel's abiding elegance and boundless sophistication are scorched into its every brick. Refined guests stroll amid the lush gardens and centuries-old courtyards, many adorned in white towelling robes, as they head for the comparative cool of the pool, where bronzed, perfect bodies lounge beguilingly on beds, or glide seamlessly through the glistening water.

Sprouts, I think. Should we have sprouts?

'You what?' says Nigel.

'Oh nothing, sorry. Didn't mean to blab out loud.'

I've texted the family and invited them all for Christmas. I'm planning the menu. Here, in the height of summer, basking on the stunning Isola di San Clemente, a short water shuttle ride from the glories of Venice, I'm contemplating Christmas. Never mind the legendary Rialto Bridge, the grandeur of the Grand Canal, the splendid Piazza San Marco, the gorgeous gondoliers. No, starters, mains, table décor and colour schemes carry more importance right now. Oh, and of course, the mandatory dilemma of the sprouts.

Hope they're not already committed, I panic. After all, this could be our last family Christmas. There's no shaking that 'could be the last time' anxiety. I'm not alone in this. We know it's irrational and yet it won't budge. As the weeks pass it becomes apparent Nigel's MND is slow. And yet none of us trust it. We're all guilty of scrambling to take photographs, desperate to capture moments with Nigel whilst we still can. There's an ill-disguised sense of urgency as we set up a perfect pose with the grandchildren, seize a chance to entrust a family grouping to eternity, take a snapshot with his siblings. Six months on, we are becoming accustomed to hiding our grief in our pockets and handbags. Ordinary conversation is back. Joyous laughter is trickling back into our lives.

The spectre of Death, however, continues to perform its role of the malevolent escort. It insists on stowing away in the suitcase and hijacking our holidays. Well, my case, for certain. It prefers my bag. I should give it a name. Something appropriate to call it when it shows up uninvited. There are many potential monikers, all unprintable.

Nigel ignores it. Since his lapse in that Estepona cove he has forbidden this encroaching menace to overshadow a single one of his remaining days. He has banished it from his thoughts. He behaves as close to normal as it is possible to do. As cheerful, gregarious, witty and full of life as ever. And, at the same time, as mindful of money. No, 'Oh to hell with it, I can't take it with me,' for him. Indeed, we are luxuriating in holidays and fabulous hotels, when considered worthy of the price tag, but the fact he is ill has not distracted him enough to inhibit his outrage at the price of the breakfast at this hotel, which means I am now adept at stealing bread buns throughout all of Venice to assuage my hunger. And once again, I am treated to a gelato instead of a gondola ride, as he is not prepared to pay the extortionate fee for a real-life glide along the canals. Nigel is still Nigel after all.

Unlike Nigel, I fail to banish the looming reality of our future from my mind. Although this pernicious presence is not so all pervading as a few weeks ago. On certain days, it lurks so deeply in the shadows I forget it's there at all. On others, it irritates, like a whingeing child kicking your seat on a plane. There are also times when I am overwhelmed. This happens when performing ordinary, insignificant activities: as I round a corner; reach for a can of beans; step out of the shower; brush my hair. Like a savage beast it leaps from its lair and punches me full in the face with such ferocity I'm knocked off my feet.

And of course, things have changed. Everything is tainted. Flawed. On our sight-seeing jaunts, when I enter an exquisite room, I no longer marvel at its magnificence. It's the crack in the ceiling that commands my attention. Where once I could delight in the breathtaking beauty of an object, a painting, a view, now, beauty is no longer without a blemish.

For me, the world's wonders have lost a little of their wonder.

11

WHERE HOPE DIES

The twenty-one storey, monolithic, concrete tower of Sheffield's Royal Hallamshire Hospital has all the charm of a neglected, eastern European, communist prison block. Equally welcoming, in the pit of the tower, is the lift lobby, which, right now, resonates with the muted grumblings of people approaching the limit of their endurance.

The overhead lights, indicating the proximity, or otherwise, of the six lifts, tantalise us trapped, intolerant folk as we agonise over which of these carriages to choose, in order to ensure our deliverance to the floor of our choice: the fifteenth, in our case.

As you might guess, we make the wrong choice and an alternative lift arrives. Mouth gaping, it spews its diverse cargo into the already crowded vestibule. Harried staff hurry to their next crisis. A pallid, scrawny young woman cautiously wheels the attached intravenous drip frame, and weaves her way to the exit to smoke one of the fags from the packet clutched in her bony hand. Visitors, relieved of their duty, scurry home, and outpatients, some appearing lost and confused, search for reassurance from the signs that they are in the right place.

'Stand back,' says Nigel, directing me away from the impatient throng surging towards the yawning doors, the perilous claustrophobia never far from the surface in the presence of crowds.

'We'll all be dead before we catch a bloody lift,' I mutter, with my customary patience.

Our hit-and-miss strategy in this lift scramble circus, developed over many months of coming here, is to head for whichever lift indicates it is the furthest away, and therefore an unattractive proposition to the uninitiated. Despite this, time and again we miss being swallowed up and doors slam shut in our faces.

Persistence rewards us at last, and the lift delivers us to the Neurology Department in this gargantuan hospital. It's usual, at this point, for me to realise I've left something important in the car. Not today, thank goodness. If I had, I swear I would take the stairs.

We park ourselves somewhere along one of the rows of pale green plastic chairs, and wait. Nigel, who could sleep in the midst of a clan of cackling hyenas, snatches a snooze, whilst I adopt the same vacant expression as my fellow zombies and gaze with lifeless eyes at the uninspiring notice boards, or, given that we're on the fifteenth floor and there's a large window, the view. Today's weather paints this panoramic, haphazard and concrete vista a dreary grey. It's one of those grimy days when the sky slouches, like an idle teenager, on the ground, and can't be arsed to lift itself up. It mirrors my mood exactly. It's this place. I hate it here. I have since the Professor killed all hope we may have cherished.

...

'Yes, it's mild MND,' she says, a well-respected leading light in the fight against MND, as she confirms the diagnosis proffered by Mr Harrop.

Mild? What does that mean? Like a little bit pregnant?

'Mild?' says Nigel.

'It's slow. And it won't change pace.'

Mild and slow? Surely this gives us hope. We could have longer than we thought. Is it like the difference between a cold and pneumonia? Meaning it won't develop into anything gross? Or does she mean mild is slow? In which case, say slow.

'Is the prognosis the same?' says Nigel, asking the precise question whirring around my head.

'Oh yes. Three to five years,' she chirps, as if sharing with us the timescale she has in mind for remaining in this particular post, before moving on to more exacting things.

'Oh, right,' says Nigel, glancing towards me, a mixture of sadness and resignation in his eyes. I reach out and take his hand in mine.

The Professor stares at us beneath arched brows and pinched lips. She has the demeanour of a boss, who, having ordered you to design the next space rocket, is flummoxed because you're still in the office. Off you trot. Run along now. She appears unaware that she has crushed the last fragment of hope, which dared to grope its way out of the locked mineshaft from where it was imprisoned. It is somehow worse hearing it for the second time, and from this instant, I loathe this place.

'How long can I expect some quality of life?' asks Nigel. A reasonable question. After all, he is new at this.

The Professor, a well-presented, intelligent woman, whose words gallop from her mouth as if to keep up with her frenetic schedule, peers at him from above the rim of her spectacles, her slim face genuinely puzzled.

'Whatever do you mean?' she says. A tad brusque, in my opinion.

Whilst expertise may run from her ears like molten lava, empathy is as remote as Saturn. Perhaps this is someone who is so focused on the disease itself, she forgets to be human. Though she understands the nuances of the motor neurones better than most, what about the myriad of emotions besieging a person when beset by a terminal illness? She's confirmed a grim diagnosis and bleak prognosis. All the decisions we make from now on will be based on her words. Any remaining ambitions Nigel hopes to achieve before he dies, he will need to do in the next three years. He might be close to death after two, and who knows if he'll make it to five? Give the man a break.

'Well, I don't know,' says Nigel, with some hesitation. 'Maybe when I could be in a wheelchair, that kind of thing,'

'Impossible to say.' Brusque, again. Train to catch? I'm going off her.

'Everybody is different. And you must appreciate, it's possible to live an acceptable quality of life when in a wheelchair.'

Her words make us squirm. Should we be ashamed for asking? How dare she scold us? We know the lives of wheelchair users are not diminished just because of the wheelchair. The image of a paralympic athlete pops into my mind and I discard it with a shake of my head. Perhaps we should apologise for not exactly looking forward to it. Still, Nigel appears to have run out of things to say and I now lack the confidence to ask any more questions.

Her expression softens. 'Do you have grandchildren?'

'Yes,' we answer in unison.

'Well, you can enjoy watching them when they visit.'

That's it. I'm off her. Nigel's a doer not a watcher. With nothing left to discuss, we escape without delay.

Later that night, as we share a bottle of wine, Nigel says, 'So, if it's slow at the outset, it will be slow at the end. When I'm fucked and can't move.'

'Yes,' I reply, having drawn the same conclusion and thought of nothing else all afternoon but the man with MND, who spent the last year of his life unable to move anything other than his eyebrows.

'We'd better make the most of now, then,' says Nigel with a grin, clinking my glass with a flourish. 'Bugger it, let's open another.'

...

This is our third visit in the research trial led by our esteemed Professor, where MND patients are administered with a dose of lithium, a substance found in batteries.

'Fancy, if all I have to do to cure this thing is suck on a battery,' said Nigel when the trial opened. If only.

We'll be here approximately three hours. Perfect timing to ensure we hit the rush hour traffic on the way home. We will see a doctor from the research team, who will interview Nigel, examine him and gauge the progression of the disease. This will be followed by blood tests, again. Questions asked last time will be asked, again. Forms completed last time, completed, again. We don't know if Nigel is taking lithium. He may be on the placebo. Still, this diligent monitoring will determine lithium's effectiveness, or otherwise, in slowing the advancement of this dreadful disease.

'You have to try,' said Nigel, when asked to participate. 'If you do nothing, you get nothing.'

So, here we are.

'Mr Casson?' calls a nurse, 'You're next.'

Next in the queue means you wait a bit further along the corridor, to the left of Reception, and opposite a chaotic anteroom housing filing-cabinets.

'There'll be a slot in there for me, soon,' laughs Nigel, pointing to a filing cabinet marked 'Deceased.'

Only you. Only you could find that funny. I punch his arm. 'You're a daft sod. You really are. Still, in spite of myself, my spirits are lifted a modicum.

An elderly man manoeuvring a mobility scooter wheels past us and stops at Reception. He hands a piece of paper to the lady behind the desk.

'Right luv,' she says in a broad South Yorkshire accent. 'Yul need sumbdy wi' yer, when yer come next week.'

'I ant got nubdy,' says the old man, his dialect so pronounced he makes the receptionist sound like the Queen.

'Wot? Nubdy?'

'Nah. Nubdy.'

'Yer must 'av sumbdy!'

'Nah. I ant. Nubdy.'

'Not nubdy?'

'That's reet, nubdy.'

'God, I love Yorkshire,' chuckles Nigel. 'Poor old bugger, he's got nubdy.'

'Wot, nubdy?' I say. 'He must 'av sumbdy!'

'Nah, nubdy.'

Our mimicry ceases as a man approaches us in a wheelchair, pushed by a nurse. His name is Matthew, a fellow MND patient we met at our last visit.

'Hi you two,' he says.

'Ey up mate,' says Nigel. 'How're you doing?'

I gasp 'Hello,' and hope the bright smile I've plastered on my face masks my shock. He was walking, albeit with a stick, at our last appointment.

'OK. Struggling to walk now though,' says Matthew, patting the wheel of the chair.

'I'm so sorry mate,' says Nigel.

'Comes to us all,' says Matthew as he is wheeled by.

'Yeah. Comes to us all,' repeats Nigel under his breath.

Will Nigel make it to the end of this trial still on his feet? Will the slices of time devoted to the trial be worthy of the sacrifice? Will it make any difference to MND's relentless approach?

12

NOT READY FOR THIS

In spite of not wishing to be members of this new gang, we're attending a meeting hosted by the MND Association. Nigel is intrigued by research currently taking place and the venue is on the doorstep, in Wetherby, the other side of York.

'It's a day out,' he says. 'Free lunch.'

Signs bearing the Association's distinct blue and orange logo direct us towards the conference room, as we enter the lobby of the three-star Days Inn Hotel. Delegates, at least a quarter of whom are in wheelchairs, are already taking their places at one of the four circular tables dominating the centre of the room. Exhibitors standing before their displays take up the space at the rear, and a stage bearing a lectern and presentation aids stands at the front. Oh no, death by PowerPoint, I groan, as I spot the OHP on the table.

A middle-aged lady, her blonde, inverted bob creating a striking contrast to her elegant navy skirt suit and red blouse, balances a clipboard on the front of her mobility scooter and greets us with an exuberant, 'Hello. Your names please?'

I oblige.

'Welcome,' she says. 'Help yourselves to refreshments and take your seats. You're at table number four. Won't be long now.'

'Do you reckon she's got it?' I say as we head for the food and beverages laid out on the table at the side.

'Yes. Why else would she be here?'

'True. Tea, coffee, or water?' I ask, while Nigel piles his plate with tuna mayo, egg mayo and classic turkey and cranberry sandwiches.

'Tea please,' he says, shoving a bite-sized piece of quiche in his mouth before adding a couple of mini pork pies to his collection.

Our plates full, we make our way to our allotted table and claim the two remaining places.

'Hi,' I say, to the table.

'Hello,' says the woman next to me. She has a bundle of biros and a pile of activity sheets with questions in bold text and empty boxes for answers. Looks like we're expected to participate. She must be the facilitator. 'Mr and Mrs Casson?' she says.

'Nigel,' mumbles Nigel.

'Julie,' I say, and add, 'and Nigel.' When he speaks it's obvious all is not well. None of the distressing ravages wrought on the body are yet evident in Nigel. Unlike our fellow delegates.

A young man, opposite, who can't be more than thirty, is breathing due only to the aid of a ventilator strapped to the back of his wheelchair. A tube from the machine, leading to the mask which covers half his face, directs the pumped air into his lungs to keep him alive. I assume, which I do a lot, the older lady seated next to him, her hand resting on the young man's arm, is his mother. There's a resemblance around the eyes extending to more than the desolation within them. She waves and introduces herself.

'Mary,' she says. 'And this is John.'

John jerks his head in greeting.

A waif of a creature, with wild, copper curls framing her face, crouches in the huge contraption of her wheelchair. It bears countless attachments, the purposes of which confound me. Her withered and twisted frame is lost in that apartment of a chair. Her hands, crooked and atrophied, lie unmoving in her lap. 'Amy,' she says, in a voice exactly like Nigel's.

A petite woman, grey hair scraped back in a simple ponytail, slices sandwiches into manageable pieces and feeds each morsel to the gaunt man seated beside her. Both his arms hang uselessly by his sides. It's disturbing and feels impertinent to stare at them. I survey the room and am confronted with a mass of disease-ravaged and broken bodies.

No way can this happen to Nigel. Not a chance. My mind can't envisage Nigel's strong, healthy muscles wasting away, his limbs becoming atrophied and helpless. My imagination won't play the video of him not breathing on his own and it's not prepared to contemplate, as he eats another sandwich, a future where he is unable to feed himself.

The food grows in my mouth and I cough the sludge into my serviette and shove it in my bag. I sip some water to stem the panic and the bile rising inside me.

'I'm not ready for this,' I whisper.

'I'm sorry,' he says, taking my hand. 'It wasn't part of the plan was it?'

I pull from his grasp, shove back my chair and flee from the room. I make it to the Ladies just as the vomit gushes from my mouth. My head remains levelled over the toilet bowl until my fear of the future is overtaken by shame. Today, for the first time, we can see what our lives will become. Sorry, Nigel says. He's sorry!

Like he's responsible somehow. And what do I do? I run. How could I? I must not run away from this. This is my world now. *Our* world. I splash my face with cold water and throw the napkin wrapped around a bit of tuna sandwich in the bin. I take a long, hard look at the woman in the mirror. The face is mine. The eyes, full of anxiety, are mine. I purse my lips and appraise that face, the way a disappointed parent considers his or her child.

'Grow up,' I say, showing her my back.

As I retake my seat, I plant a kiss on Nigel's head and I whisper, 'Love you.'

He grins at me and takes my hand. This time I do not pull away. The next thirty minutes are spent completing the activity sheets, brainstorming how the MNDA could support the carers of those with MND. Our ideas will inform the library of resources the association provides to help people like us, like these people here, their carers and families, all plunged into the devastating world of MND.

What was their world before MND? What careers did they follow? What hobbies and passions did they pursue? How bravely have they dealt with their loss? All the while their bodies are destroyed by MND, their personalities remain the same. They retain the likes, loves and irritations that shaped them and made them who they are. Here in this room, surrounded by those whose fortunes we now share, I understand how difficult it is to appreciate the person behind the broken body and unintelligible speech, until you adopt the guise of the invalid yourself. When you do, it is humbling.

MND was first diagnosed by a French physician, J M Charcot, in 1874. The origin is still unknown. A cure, still out of reach. What scientists, researchers and medical professionals know, is equal to what they don't. They can tell us with authority what is happening inside the body, how the motor neurones should function and what happens as they die. Yet beating this thing continues to mystify the scientific arena. Despite constant fundraising activities, those aiming to unravel the enigma are thwarted by lack of money. The 5000 people with MND at any one time in the UK are simply not enough to attract the millions it will demand to develop a cure. As the presentation concludes, the delegates in the room are left in no doubt a cure will not be found in time for them. Even so, those involved in the fight won't give up. And therefore, hope exists. Hope for others. Hope for the future.

Before leaving, we subscribe to the MNDA's quarterly magazine *Thumb Print* and buy a dozen *Thumbs Up* lapel pins, the symbol of hope inspired by the final gesture made by David Niven, who died of MND in 1983. Was it an optimistic gesture of hope? I wonder. Or was his thumb the only thing he could still move?

We browse the exhibitors until Nigel stops, fascinated by a piece of equipment with the potential to eradicate everybody's worst nightmare. Who amongst us doesn't shudder at the thought of being unable to wipe our own bum? Here, with the ability to prolong independence and maintain dignity, is a toilet that washes and dries the user. No need for hands. A simple, yet life-enhancing object.

'Put that on the must-have list,' he says.

13

OUR SPANISH LOVE AFFAIR

April 2008

Who could have imagined, twenty-three years and nine jobs ago, that MND would end my career and drive me from the college? Still, unlike so many senior managers I've witnessed bullied from the building, there's no fist shoving me in the back. Few college managers survive the turbulent macho management style currently dominating FE. Most clash with an incoming Principal at some point and, following a little gun-to-the-head persuasion, disappear faster than a gambler's chips. Career over.

My own years here have not been without friction. Infuriating decisions and misguided strategies, in my opinion, have at times led to taxing episodes, where the compulsion to storm out of the building in a huff, slamming the door behind me, has threatened to triumph over the need to earn a few quid. I've locked myself in the loo and contemplated principle over pay, more than once.

I trudge across the foyer for the final time, clutching the bouquet of flowers the few members of staff just presented me with – its perfume struggling to dilute the unrivalled aromas of pot noodles, teenage feet and mucky mop swished across dusty wood. The kind words from my boss and a couple of my closest colleagues replay in my mind: the challenges we've faced over the years, our accomplishments, a funny story or two, the earnest promises to stay in touch.

I remember my first day – my first part-time teaching job. Nigel was late collecting me from home and sped towards the college like his truck was packed with stolen diamonds, instead of bags of scaffold fittings, boards and tubes, rattling like an improvising skiffle band. He swung the truck into the car park and hurtled round the mini-roundabout so violently I expected one of the 21 footers to fly like a javelin from the rear and launch itself right through the window into this very foyer.

'Do well, darling,' he said. I'll pick you up at nine.'

'Sod off. You've made me late.'

Jumping from the wagon I feared I'd ripped the slit of my smart black pencil skirt to an embarrassing level, and tottered on my agonising, patent stilettos towards the main door. Eighties perm, matching bright red lips and nails, liberal quantities of Armani Code to disguise the stink of nicotine and the coffee I'd earlier spilled on my jacket, should all combine to portray a professional young woman launching a promising career. Or so I thought.

Twenty-three years later, here I am, retiring at forty-nine. My departure could not be more unexpected or unwelcome.

'It could be worse,' says Nigel. 'We could be skint.'

Not kidding. How difficult would it be if I had no choice but to continue to work? And how distressing would it be for Nigel, if his partner hadn't supported him by running the business without him? When not knocking a few shots off his round, Nigel has been enjoying harassing the insurance company handling his critical illness claim.

'I'm dying,' he says to the unfortunate assistant on the line, exaggerating his already alarming voice.

'What if you didn't tick the MND box?' I say. 'Did you specify all possible illnesses?' 'How could anybody anticipate MND?'

Yes, he ticked the box. He ticked them all. He's not daft. He wouldn't presume the only illnesses likely to blight a scaffolder would be restricted to injuries sustained from falling off a scaffold. His pestering succeeded, the insurance company paid out swiftly and freed me from the obligation to work.

Now, someone else will be required to fulfill my latest role of Quality Manager. I don't envisage a frantic scramble for the post: it's not the sexiest of jobs. A significant chunk of time is spent re-inventing the wheel, churning out procedures to replace comparable procedures with an amended but similar title, hoping the new ones will do a far better job. Impose said procedures on the long-suffering staff, then follow up by crawling all over them conducting compliance audits. No, the job will be dumped on some poor sod with a thousand other things to do.

The college doors swing closed behind me and I glance up at the four-storey glass and steel structure. I've had an office on every floor. I am going to miss this place: the students, the teachers, my colleagues. I march towards my car, alone. No fanfare. No regrets. No tears.

It is time to move on. Time for Nigel and me to relish our remaining days together. Nigel's modest bucket list is now complete. His shiny, golden coloured S-type Jaguar, complete with cream leather seats and walnut dash, purrs like its living namesake, as it awaits its master's pleasure.

Its master's pleasure is to luxuriate in a leisurely drive to southern Spain, the region we vowed to revisit, and are already half in love with. Located between San Pedro de Alcantara and Estepona is a select, gated urbanisation of twelve three-bedroomed, spacious dwellings, arranged amidst nurtured gardens and encircling an impressive pool. El Paraiso – paradise – our home for the next eight months, could not be more delightfully situated, nestled as it is within a proficient three-wood's reach of two spectacular golf courses. Not for Nigel the stress of dashing to all points on the planet in pursuit of the places he hasn't yet visited. No, he wishes to wallow for a while in the Andalucía way.

'Life is too short to rush it,' he says.

We plan to explore this vibrant land in our golden carriage. We may even have a stab at learning the language.

Felices Fiestas!

...

Once I've scrubbed the walls of our new home free of previous occupants' fingerprints, I learn from the local property-come-maintenance manager, he intended to repaint it. Marvellous. No matter, it needed cleaning anyway. I like to remove the muck of strangers before replacing it with our own.

Once cleaned, we settle into our sun-soaked home. Our mornings are spent lingering over a healthy breakfast of fruit, freshly squeezed orange juice, toast, perhaps an egg or two, enjoyed on the opulent terrace. Here we are entertained by the striking hoopoe birds, adorned with their distinctive crown of orange feathers, as they dance upon our lawn.

In the afternoons, we play out. Sometimes, golf is our game of choice. I thrash around the course in pursuit of a par, whilst Nigel eats it up like a pro, sinking putts and striking the fairways like Jack Nicklaus giving a masterclass. Because we're kids from the fifties, we frequently straddle our new, if not stylish, bicycles in pursuit of adventures so thrilling it would make Tintin's exploits look tedious.

'What d'ya reckon? Shall we buy 'em?' says Nigel as we are stocking up on supplies in the mammoth El Cortes Ingles, a hypermarket selling a consummate array of goods from paperclips to four-poster beds.

I whip around from the wine aisle to find Nigel, beaming like a kid on Christmas morning, holding aloft two pushbikes, one in each hand, as though each weighed no more than a pack of sugar.

'Are you insane?'

'They're only seventy-five euros apiece,' he continues. 'Bargain.'

'Top quality then,' I groan, saddlesore already. 'I can't remember when I last rode a bike.'

'That's why we should buy 'em. It'll be great.'

'How will we fit them in the car,' I protest, searching for a reason to leave them right here in the shop. 'How do we organise delivery?' I'm the one who has to do all the talking and I wouldn't know where to begin. 'What the hell is the Spanish word for bike?'

'Calm down,' he says. 'I'll squeeze them in the car.'

He does. No problem.

In fact, the bikes prove to be one of Nigel's inspired purchases. Once you've mastered the juggling act of lugging the damn thing up the steel steps and over the footbridge which crosses the notorious Autovia del Mediterraneo, you discover a world you would never happen upon by car and to which you would never venture on foot.

We peek through hedges into the private and exquisite gardens of the luxury villas lining the beach. We nose our way around neighbouring communities to compare them with our own. We skirt the boundaries of championship golf courses and declare our intention to return with clubs, in order to challenge that which looks easy from a bike, and we jiggle into beach bar after beach bar.

One cycling expedition takes us to the door of a modest independent school offering Spanish classes to ex pats. Instead of hurtling straight past the place, we enrol and book ourselves in for two private lessons a week.

'Typical,' I say to Nigel, as we arrive at our first session, jotters, pens and gleaming new Collins Spanish Dictionary tucked into a rucksack on Nigel's now, gingerbread brown, back.

'*Que?*' he says.

'You struggle to speak English, so you choose to learn Spanish?'

'*Si!*'

He ties the bikes to the railings and waves at Maria, our teacher, who is standing in the doorway, waiting to greet us.

'*Hola! Que tal?*' he says, like a native, before dashing for the door in full teacher's pet mode.

'Bloody show-off,' I say, following on behind, so giddy with pride I suspect I might cry.

Maria, whilst enthusiastic, is all over the place with her lesson planning. No matter how many hours I spend practising, conjugating verbs and drilling vocabulary, without some focused reinforcement exercises, we will never become as accomplished in this fascinating tongue as I would like.

'She needs to give us specific tasks to do between classes, so we review our progress next time and build on it,' I say, while sunbathing in the garden and attempting to grind the words '*naranjas,*' '*zanahorias*' and '*chicharos*' into my memory.

'What you on about?' says Nigel, from his lounger, slumber not far away.

'Well, we're learning vocabulary for fruit and vegetables. She could send us to the supermarket, instruct us to make our list in Spanish, speak to the check-out operators in nothing other than Spanish, report back on how much it cost, in Spanish. You know, stuff like that.'

'So bugger off to the supermarket.'

'Mmm,' I say, deflated. 'Fair one.'

'Julie, you're not at work anymore. Lighten up.'

I close the book on the fruit and veg chapter as Nigel's gentle snoring tells me he's asleep. 'You're right,' I say to my snoozing husband, and, to the vivid orange hoopoe bird, flickering like a flame amongst the crimson bougainvillea, I add, 'I could make her a far better teacher though.' He's not listening either.

The Spanish classes are at least beneficial for our livers as they keep us away from our favourite beach bar for a few hours, where Nigel recites his newly acquired language skills for Raoul, our polite and patient waiter.

Considerable time is spent exploring places in anticipation of family visits, an advance party on a mission to compile a must see and do list.

'Who's coming next,' says Nigel, as we drop Paula and Tom off at Malaga Airport, following their week's holiday.

'Mel and Derek on the fifteenth. Les and Sally two weeks later. Tracey's flying over from Tenerife later in June.'

'Bloody popular all of a sudden, aren't we?'

'Certainly are,' I say, waving as Paula and Tom disappear into the departure terminal. 'I'm a holiday rep.'

'You're OK with it, though aren't you?' says Nigel, steering the car away from the airport. 'All the visitors? Not too much work for you?'

'Are you kidding? I'm loving it.'

'Brilliant,' he says, patting my hand. 'I'm grateful you know, for everything you're doing.'

The seat belt prevents me from reaching over to kiss his cheek, so I stroke his face instead and let my hand rest on his shoulder.

'Don't be daft. I'm having the time of my life.'

'Me too,' he says, before adding. 'When are the kids coming?'

'Ellie and Danny and boys are here for three weeks in the school holidays. And Becky of course. House full.'

'Perfect,' he says, easing the sleek golden Jag onto the shimmering AP-7 motorway.

I close my eyes and, like all dedicated holiday reps, conjure up a shedload of stimulating activities with which to delight our forthcoming guests. Over the next few months, whether by car, bicycle or on foot, we traverse the entirety of this sun-soaked province, and in so doing, develop a deep and enduring affection for this Spanish gem. Of the palaces of Granada, the battlements of Cadiz, the patios of Cordoba and the bodegas of Jerez, along with all the sparkling cities and ancient white pueblos in between, we will never tire.

We immerse ourselves in the magical, endless festivals where the zealous Spaniards frolic to pulsating music, all night long. Mesmerising, raven-haired flamenco dancers illuminate every street corner, the swirling gowns, stamping feet and clicking castanets telling their passionate and tragic story to the haunting wail of the Spanish guitar. We eat paella from a gigantic *paellera*, designed to serve five hundred revellers, and we are engulfed in a maelstrom of energy and fun.

It isn't difficult to develop a penchant for tapas and a love of sardines cooked atop charcoal on the beach, washed down with plenty of sangria. Lingering lunches lead to lazy siestas, before the beguiling chiringuitos and the smooth, calming rhythms of chill-out music call us to dinner and beyond.

The global financial crisis doesn't dent this idyllic existence. It is one of the happiest times of our lives. Our old antagonist: Death, given to hijacking our holidays, remains mostly hidden, emerging, on occasion, from the bottom of a bottle of gin.

But it is time to leave.

The lock slots into place as Nigel rotates the key in the front door for the final time. The Jag, engine already running, glistens in the glowering heat, whilst the gentle hum of the air conditioner cools the interior. It waits at the end of the path, impatient to be off.

Nigel reluctantly steers the car away from this parcel of paradise and up to the top of the hill, where just last week, I tumbled off my bike as we staggered home from one of our adventures. Too much gin in the sangria I suspect.

The doors are closing on this episode of our lives. A new door is opening. MND is marching through it, and we must prepare.

14

TWO STEPS AHEAD

Nigel's body lurches six inches off the operating table, as the surgeon stabs him in the stomach. A nurse, meanwhile, rams a tube down his throat. The ensuing sound is like a mugger suffocating an angry dog.

'Tell him to stop,' I yell, from behind the glass screen, in the corner of the operating theatre.

Karen, our nurse from the hospice, the one responsible for granting Nigel's wish that I observe this horror, rests her hand on my shoulder and says, 'It's alright Julie, he's in capable hands.'

'What? He's in agony. I can't bear to listen.' I cover my ears to blot out Nigel's desperate retching.

'He's sedated. He's fine. It's all part of the procedure.'

I used to like Karen. I'm changing my mind. This procedure, this insertion of the PEG, or feeding tube, is, according to Karen, a sensible idea. Indeed, she hasn't failed to mention its merits on any one of her monthly visits.

'It gives you options,' she says, time and again. 'Should you lose the ability to swallow. At least you'll be fed through the tube.'

'Better than starving to death,' says Nigel, as her gentle persistence nudges closer to victory.

'Yes,' she says. 'Although the procedure must be carried out sooner, rather than later, as you need the strength to endure it.'

Sounds pretty bloody ghastly to me. But Nigel is persuaded and here we are. Having replaced Vanessa, who, as we know, is busy doing a spot of God-bothering, Karen has supported us now for almost a year. Mid-thirties, married to a chap called Ian, mum to a four-year-old son, whom she adores. A vegetarian, yet lives on a farm, does not possess a TV, cropped, no need for a brush, fair hair, Christmas apple cheeks brightening a pale make-up-less face and, I bet she wears wellies teamed with flowery frocks when she's not adorned in black trousers, easy on, easy off loafers and a practical M&S jumper.

'Well done, Mr Casson,' says the surgeon to my now silent husband, his battered body, exhausted and inert. 'All finished. That went well.'

'Come on Julie,' says Karen. 'Let's move him to the hospice.'

At last. Let's escape this hell hole.

Nigel enjoys undisturbed slumber during the wait for the ambulance, and doesn't stir when he is transported from Scarborough Hospital to a room at St Catherine's Hospice, and enough morphine to level an elephant reunites him with oblivion when he is transferred from trolley to bed.

Our home for the next seventy-two hours is a simple room, with profiling bed in the centre, upon which Nigel dreams drug-induced dreams. Next to the bed is a riser recliner, covered in blue corduroy fabric. Fabric. Why fabric and not leather? Far easier to clean. There's a matching blue corduroy futon upon which I am supposed to sleep. Doubtful, given the lumps. At least they're not the usual pink or bloody green. A pocket-sized TV hangs from a wall mount, its screen set at an angle to catch the sun, and also the dust the cleaner has failed to remove.

As you might expect, there is a well-equipped wetroom with walk-in and roll-in shower. Reminds me of home and our soon to be completed wetrooms. I study the detail. Don't want to forget anything important. It's possible to hang the sink at the usual height or lower to suit a wheelchair user. Better decide what's best for Nigel. The toilet is raised on a three-inch platform, easy on and off access, I suppose, although Nigel's already determined he's having the no hands needed, wash and dry your bum, loo. Grab rails are in abundance. We'll choose smarter chrome ones for home, not these white plastic bars. A shower chair on wheels is parked in the shower area. Don't need one of those yet. Ah, a ceiling hoist with a track running from shower to toilet. Hadn't thought of that. Must mention to Gary to ensure the ceiling in the wetroom will support a hoist and Nigel's weight. Bet Nigel's already told him, given his expertise in construction surpasses mine. Perhaps it won't come to that. He may never need a ceiling hoist. The way Karen talks you'd expect him to drop down dead right now. Still, better to be prepared, Nige says, like the cute boy scout he claims he once was. DYB, DYB, DYB, and all that.

Whilst Nigel sleeps on, I slip outside and I'm delighted to discover the patio doors open onto a quadrangle, each room having its own neat, private terrace. In the centre, a charming garden boasts a manicured lawn, bordered on all sides with a mixture of fuchsia shrubs, alabaster and salmon pink hydrangea, golden roses and violet lavender. It's a balmy, late September day. The autumn sunshine floods this picturesque courtyard and soothes with its mellow warmth.

'How lovely,' I say, taking a seat on the painted wooden bench outside the room. Enjoying this tranquil place I close my eyes and rest my head against the wall behind me. The caress of the sun on my face, the whisper of the breeze as it kisses my cheek, the cheerful chirruping of the birds as they flit amongst the plants transport me to Spain. Oh, how I wish we could go back there. What a wonderful time we had. Impossible, I know. Our suitcases are packed away, our travels over. I scold myself for longing for the unattainable. We've enjoyed three spectacular years since Nigel's diagnosis, and, against all predictions, he's still on his feet. Just. Most people with MND would be dead by now. I should be grateful. I am grateful. I am.

I'm also grateful Nigel is the man he is. He has taken charge of this disease and is determined to stay two steps ahead of it. Not one step. Two. Nothing will sneak up on Nigel. Nothing and nobody. Perhaps his time in Northern Ireland trained him to anticipate danger, like the attack of the gunman, shielded by the rioters, waiting for the parting of the crowds for his moment to fire. Always the first to throw a punch when a drunken brawl threatens, Nigel ends the fight before it kicks off.

'Drive as though everybody else on the road is an idiot,' he'd say, when teaching me to drive. 'Predict what might happen and be ready to avoid it.' He said the same to the kids. Strange how he's been the victim or protagonist of more road accidents than the rest of us.

'It's all about control,' he says. 'I won't let this disease take over.'

Realistic and practical, accepting of the unstoppable progress of MND, he is determined to control as many elements of his life as is feasible. He will be ready for it. Each new development will be expected, and prepared for, in that he will ensure he has all the equipment in place to support his physical needs.

'I won't wait until I can't walk, before I order a wheelchair,' he says, 'I'll make sure I'm two steps ahead.'

'Ha ha. Funny.'

His two-steps challenge includes Nigel's bag of death, the concoction of injectable drugs designed to relieve end-of-life torment, stored in the kitchen cupboard, waiting for its moment. It may well be nudging its use by date.

'It makes sense to keep a stock at home,' says Karen. 'Then you're ready. And there's a bank holiday coming up.'

'Am I likely to die before Tuesday?' says Nigel, enjoying himself. He loves to tease her. Karen's quiet steadfastness amuses him.

'I bet you were a Girl Guide, weren't you?' he says, as Karen recommends additional, be prepared, strategies to ensure Nigel's ultimate demise is as he would wish.

'I was, as a matter of fact,' she says.

No surprise there. Indeed, not only was Karen a Girl Guide, but also reached the rank of Sixer, whatever that is, and this childhood character development enabled her to achieve the accolade of the Duke of Edinburgh's Gold Award. Her well-deserved pride makes those Christmas apple cheeks glow ever rosier.

'Reassuring to know I'm in safe hands,' says Nigel.

All this may explain Karen's approach to her 'things to do list'. She has succeeded in encouraging Nigel to complete a 'Do Not Resuscitate Directive' and 'Advanced Care Plan' which declares Nigel will not receive treatment or medication merely for the purpose of prolonging life. Simply put, he does not want to be taken to hospital, nor does he wish to be revived. Once completed,

Karen hands these instructions to me, folded inside a white plastic container, sporting a green cross.

'You need to keep these in the fridge,' she says.

'What?'

'Everybody has a fridge,' she says. 'And, should anything happen, all attending medical professionals know to look in the fridge.'

'Right, I understand,' I say, popping the container inside the fridge door.

'And here's a green cross sticker to fix on the outside,' she says. 'Then they'll know which cupboard is the fridge.'

You're having a laugh, I think, as I take the sticker from her hand. This glorious new kitchen hasn't yet had chance to gather dirt. Can you begin to contemplate how, like a shameless hussy, I prostituted myself to persuade Nigel to add a new kitchen to the renovation plan? Not until I came up with the brilliant idea of replacing a whole wall with glass doors leading straight out onto the patio – like Spain – did he relent. While it broke my heart to part with our battered old pine table, this uber modern island is worth the waterfall of tears. I run my fingers along the gleaming worktop of my beloved island until I reach the sparkling, seamless, integrated, kitchen sink. Weeks it took to find the right one. And, as for the tap adorning it, can you believe how much it cost? These are not simply cupboards plonked around a room. The design, style and arrangement of this *furniture,* its delicate cream complexion contrasting superbly with the arresting damson hue embellishing the walls, unite in their depiction of a distinctive creation, inspiring the invention of all manner of culinary delights. Do you expect me to blemish the smooth, faultless exterior of my integrated appliance by sticking a green cross on it? Not a bloody chance.

'Of course,' I say.

My reflections are interrupted by a commotion at the opposite side of the quadrangle. I open my eyes and watch as a patient is wheeled out onto the terrace. Two nurses pull at the foot of a bed, whilst a lady, who I recognise as Hannah, our occupational therapist, on account of her exceptional height, pushes the bed into a sunny spot. She sees me and waves. I wave back, intrigued.

A man, mid-forties I guess, is inclined in the bed, propped against a cloud of pillows. His flesh is so shrunken the ridges of his shoulder blades are visible through the white T-shirt hanging from his body. Gossamer thin skin stretched against sharp cheekbones protrude from a grey sunken face. One of the nurses protects his bald head with a baseball cap. Hannah disappears into the room and emerges with an acoustic guitar, the body of which she places on the man's lap before plumping the pillows around him. Long, bony fingers reach for and adjust the tuning pegs whilst his other hand strums at the frets until he's satisfied. He tips the peak of his cap, acknowledging his audience. He rests his head against the pillows and plays.

The haunting melody of Eric Clapton's *Tears in Heaven* permeates through this enchanting courtyard like the soft murmur of angels. The mild, stirring breeze ceases its purring and the harmonious spotted breasted thrush stills its song. I close my eyes and surrender myself to the magic of the moment, savouring each mournful note as the music seeps through the pores of my skin into my soul. The garden holds its breath. We listen. Captivated.

All too soon, it is over. The musician, this talented guitarist, is exhausted. As his fingers fall from the frets of his instrument, a darkening shadow obscures the sun and a sudden breeze whips the garden awake once more. Hannah and the two nurses wheel the man back into the room in which he will, in the days ahead, undoubtedly die. Unlike Nigel, he will not be going home.

Nigel is awakening as I enter from the terrace.

'Did I hear guitar playing?' he says, his voice groggy from morphine.

'You did, yes.'

'I thought I was dreaming. Clapton wasn't it?'

'Not him personally,' I say.

'No kidding.'

'Yes, it was magical.' I place a tender kiss on his forehead. 'How are you feeling?'

'Awful. Everything hurts. And I need a piss.'

'I'll find help.'

I'm in luck. There are two nurses on duty at the nurses' station. I assume they're nurses, although they're wearing different uniforms. The one in the dark blue tunic, stocky, five-foot-five-ish, is clearly in charge and seems familiar. The other, younger and petite, wears a mint green tabard. Both are free to help.

'Do we need a wheelchair?' asks mint green.

'Oh, I don't know.'

'We'll manage,' says dark blue. 'Come on.'

Nigel is attempting to lift himself up in bed when we arrive back at the room. 'Hurry up.'

'Right, let's have you,' says dark blue. 'Oh, hello you. How's the golf?'

Ah ha, that's where I've seen her. Golf club. Incapable of chit-chat, Nigel responds with an unintelligible grunt and a nod of recognition. Nigel is a heavy man weighing around thirteen and a half stone, yet dark blue hauls him up and swings his legs over the side of the bed like he's a mere child. She orders him to slip one arm over her shoulder, the other over teeny mint green's, who I now know, having read her name badge, is Sheila. Between them, they ease Nigel off the bed. When his feet hit the carpet, he yelps as if dunked in a vat of molten lava.

'Come on, you can do it,' says dark blue. 'One step at a time. We've got you.'

If I wasn't witnessing this, I would never believe these two women, of opposing height and build, painful wobble though it is, could make it to the toilet, bearing Nigel's weight on their shoulders, in the way they do. No wonder nurses suffer from bad backs. I spring like a lame gazelle from one foot to another, as if I'm the one desperate for the loo. I trot along behind in case I could be the slightest bit of help should they drop him.

'I don't know how you do it,' I say, once Nigel is ensconced in the wetroom.

'You get used to it,' says dark blue, Sharon, according to her name badge. 'Has anyone shown you how to clean the PEG yet?'

'PEG?'

'The gastrostomy tube.'

'Oh, I see,' I say, unaccustomed to the term. 'No.'

'Ok, I'll show you when he's back in bed.'

The journey back to bed isn't anything like as smooth as the trip to the toilet. This time, Nigel cries in anguish with each torturous step he is forced to take. He howls in protest as the pain rips his belly apart. Wretched, shuddering and broken, he collapses into bed. Sharon despatches Sheila in search of a doctor and within minutes, the phenomenon of morphine has once again worked its magic. Cleaning of the PEG must wait.

Later, when the garden is shrouded in the September gloom, when the doctors' rounds are complete and a profound hush has descended upon the hospice, I curl up in the corduroy blue riser recliner, Kindle in hand, TV switched on, volume muted, listening to the steady whisp and rhythm of Nigel's calm, drug-induced breathing.

Karen pops in to see us. 'How's he doing?' she whispers.

'He's quiet now. Zonked until morning, I hope.'

'Excellent.' She hands me a glass containing a translucent liquid, straw, ice and a slice of lemon. 'I've brought you this. Thought you could do with a G and T.'

'There's a bar?' I say, taking the glass in astonishment.

'We keep a stock for emergencies,' she says. 'And you've had a rough day.'

'Wow! Thank you.'

'You're welcome,' she says, heading for the door. 'Hope your night is peaceful. I'll call on you both tomorrow.'

I settle back in the chair and swallow a third of the cool, refreshing gin and tonic in one greedy gulp. God, that's amazing. This place is full of surprises.

And as for Karen? Well, I always did like her.

15

MND DECLARES WAR

The purplish-blue veins in his neck are taut as cheese wire. Teeth, exposed between pared lips and clamped like a wild dog at a rabbit, fail to contain the hissing rasp of each ragged breath. Shoulders stooped, arms juddering as though shot through with a thousand volts, Nigel stabs the walking aid along the corridor in faltering jerks, as he battles with every quaking muscle in his treacherous body, to haul one sluggish foot in front of the other.

'Wheelchair?' I call from the hallway.

He stops. The attempt to force a path through cloying concrete draws to a sensible close. His breathing calms. He grunts his assent.

'You push yourself too hard, Nig.'

'Maybe. But you've gotta fight.'

'Have you? You're not in the army now, you know.'

'No,' he says, dropping into the chair with a bump. 'Can't stop fighting.'

'OK you stubborn bugger. But I bet even your old boss, the Duke of Boots, knew when to back off.'

'Bollocks,' he says, nudging the chair's control to its highest speed. 'Onward!' he yells, zooming off into the lounge, victory fist punching the air. 'Make us a cuppa, will you?'

'You win,' I whisper to his departing back. 'For now. But how soon before you lose?'

Filling the kettle, I pause to admire the sparkling new, monobloc tap, which, as I tell myself daily, I must protect from the damaging effects of Scarborough's limescale-ridden water. Obsessing over trivia is becoming a habit. It's so comforting to revel in the preoccupation of planning a new kitchen, choosing tiles for wetrooms, agonising over which sanitary ware provokes the grandest 'wow,' contemplating which shower head, which screen, which bloody grab rail does the job better than any other. All preferable to focusing on the unrelenting attack on Nigel's limbs.

MND slithers like a slug in the night. Starting with the odd stumble here and there, caused by the distinct weakness in Nigel's left leg. As a stylish fellow, this encumbrance is addressed with the aid of one of his elegant canes, topped with a choice of snake, crown, or golf club head. However, they're not up to the job for long. The canes are now assigned to the porch, along with the umbrellas. Next, comes the walker, on loan from the equipment centre. No point buying one. And, as Nigel will always prepare for the inevitable, we accept the offer of an indoor electric wheelchair.

Expecting the inevitable doesn't suppress the shock when it transpires. We know MND is advancing, yet we remain helpless, as the disease deploys its army of destroyers throughout Nigel's body, the initial battalion marching towards his legs. The objective is to carry out a perpetual, violent assault on the muscles. The first wave thrusts at them until weakened by incessant twitching. The next surge batters the already disabled prey, until brutalised by never-ending seizures. Countless reinforcements prolong the onslaught without mercy, until, defeated and broken, the muscles surrender to paralysis and die.

Like Generals stationed at the perimeter of the battlefield, we witness the execution of this combat beneath Nigel's skin. What begins as a tremulous quivering, like a plague of scurrying insects trapped below the surface, become ripples of serpents swirling in a riotous, alien sea.

'We will defeat you,' the assailant mocks. 'These legs won't work much longer mate.'

Defenceless and battle weary, legs locked in spasm, Nigel retreats to the safety of the wheelchair.

Meanwhile, platoons of special forces are secreted throughout his body. Shoulders, arms, chest, hands, neck, tongue. Camps are established. Weapons made ready. Troops dig in and await the command. They advance with stealth, in silence, reaching the target undetected. Raids occur when he's sleeping, watching TV, reading the paper. This is not ferocious plundering, this is steady, sadistic sabotage.

Signs of approaching victory emerge during the campaign: the morning Nigel no longer has the strength to hold up his head without the support of a neck brace; the day two hands, not one, are needed to grasp his cup of tea; the inability to drink without the aid of a straw. The ever-increasing call on aids such as the mobile hoist, now the sole means of transferring Nigel's body from chair or bed, heralds the disease's ultimate triumph.

As his weakened body becomes the prison from which there will be no release, and with the realisation the restrictions imposed by this incarceration will worsen until he's able to do nothing for himself, Nigel is engulfed by an alarming new vulnerability.

Denied the intuitive fight or flight response to peril, this intolerable defencelessness triggers severe panic attacks: his breath quickens, trapped in his throat; his hands shake and his body drips with sweat; he glares, with fearful eyes, at some imaginary demon and he is unable to speak. We can do nothing to help and Lorazepam has no impact.

This, more than physical disability, is for Nigel, the greater enemy.

16
DON'T FORGET ME

Like dawn mist swirling above a freezing lake, the people we once were, dissolve, along with the dwindling spectre of the life we shared. Reluctant to leave, we cling like leeches to our fortifications of familiarity, dragging ourselves to the Indigo as often as we can. We frequent the handful of restaurants in Scarborough where wheelchair access is possible. When overpowered by physical challenges, we host pub nights at home, where family and friends gather to enjoy drinks, pub grub, and amiable banter. Ironically, the harmonious buzz of happy chatter only increases Nigel's mounting isolation.

Nigel's speech, in particular, the formation of sounds, is not worsening. In fact, Craig says, 'Dad's speech is improving.' It isn't. That's an illusion. The truth is, we are much better listeners. If anything, his speech is slower. No longer is he first to lead the banter with a speedy retort, injecting effortless wit into the mix. By the time he draws breath and opens his mouth to contribute, the topic is way ahead of him. So, pub nights are over, socialising with friends is restricted to two at a time and restaurants are not on the menu.

As a result, our lives are transformed. Long, mundane days are spent at home. The busy couple we used to be, capable of cramming a thousand tasks into twenty-four hours, now devote great chunks of the morning to ruminating over the *Yorkshire Post's* cryptic crossword. The TV, once a silent anathema in the corner, tolerated exclusively on Sunday evenings – the one night of the week we would venture into the lounge – is now permitted to bore us with programmes like *Homes under the Hammer* and *Heir Hunters*.

Paradoxically, the contracting reality of Nigel's world is expanding into the virtual one, through Facebook and the net. Many hours are devoted to online poker and his jokes reach more friends now than ever before. On those precious days when the sun shines, we wander along the Esplanade, Nigel parks his chair at the end of a bench and we linger for a short while, delighting in the spectacular panorama of Scarborough's South Bay.

On the whole, we replace frustration with patience. We cherish the monotony of routine and expect nothing from the day. We are successful, for the most part, in avoiding the temptation to obscure our present by obsessing about our future. We know the future. The Grim Reaper is camping on our doorstep and we're in no hurry to open the door and let him in.

Still, there are moments when it's impossible not to mourn the past.

'Don't forget me, will you?' says Nigel from nowhere.

I retrieve the empty cup from his outstretched hand. 'Forget you?'

'Yes, the man I used to be.'

His arm flops onto his lap and, resting his head on the back of the recliner, his tired eyes, smudged with loss, bore into mine.

'Not a chance,' I say, placing a kiss on his forehead.

'I miss me,' he says, his voice no more than a whisper.

For a second, I'm speechless. Submitting to melancholy is so unlike him. The cheerful disposition with which he greets each new debilitating development inspires the rest of us to cope. We are left chastened by his positivity. So much so, that on those self-indulgent days, when all I can do is crawl behind the settee and cry my heart out, I am compelled to stick a stencil of a smile on my face, choke back the tears and swallow the lump in my throat.

'I miss us,' I say.

He reaches for my hand but the effort crushes him and his arm flops onto the chair. 'I love you,' he says. 'Don't forget that either.'

'Never,' I say. 'I will never forget you. And I will always love you, no matter what.'

'Thank you,' he says, his eyes closing.

'No need to thank me,' I say. 'Now, off to sleep while I prepare tea. When you wake up, we'll find a soppy film on the telly and have a bloody good boo.'

'Great idea.'

Forget him? Inconceivable.

I grab the potatoes from the pantry and commence peeling. I won't forget you Nigel. But will others? Our grandchildren may already have forgotten how things used to be. Jemma and Amy especially, still so young, may suppose you always had a wheelchair and a strange, scary voice. Whilst Ben and Tom still recall the fun they had with you, time will steal their memories as surely as it will steal you.

MND gnaws at its victim like a rat eating garbage. A tiny bit more vanishes every day. Bit by bit, Nigel, MND has robbed you of your strength and your body. And far worse, it has robbed you of your sense of self. Will it stop there? Or will it seep into your soul and claim your spirit? Will your optimism and sense of fun fade as disappointment and despair become your constant companions? How tempting must it be, when forced to adopt the clumsy guise of the invalid, to disappear to a safe and unchallenging place? It must be easier to shrink into the seclusion of the shadows, seeking refuge in the comforting fog of invisibility, than it is to battle incessantly with an unbeatable enemy. The deeper you retreat into the fog, the harder it is for others to find you. The harder it is to remember. Nigel, you never vanished into the fog. You would not permit it to swathe you in its shroud and I haven't lost you yet. You are still you. I may not recall the timbre of your voice before MND retuned it, but there is much I will always treasure and lots I'll never forget.

Our first date. How the butterflies leapt in my stomach as we held hands on the bus to Bradford. How we both wore brown suits and the pairing made me giddy. Like it was meant to be. You took me to a pub mooted to welcome IRA sympathisers. You, with your cropped hair, the essence of a squaddie not long home from Belfast. I fell in love with you right there and then.

What about the first night we stayed up until dawn, so intent on discovering each other we couldn't let the evening end? We greeted the sunrise by walking in the long grass, dowsed with morning dew. Everyone should walk in the long grass at least once.

Enshrined in my memory is the time you worked on Barden Chambers in Leeds, supporting the face of the building with scaffolding. You knew what time I would round the corner from the bus station, on my way to work. There you were, hanging upside down like a chimpanzee, waving your arms and showing off. There was no way I could miss you.

'That's my boyfriend,' I said to the fella who travelled with me on the bus and accompanied me to Greek Street. I marvelled as you leapt from lift to lift like a mountain goat, throwing those heavy boards around with the ease and precision of a champion archer firing arrows at a target.

'Isn't he amazing?' I said, entranced.

Whatshisname raised his eyebrows and harrumphed. Bet he thought you were mad. I suspect he was jealous. I fell deeper in love with you that morning.

When I think how we fretted over that bank loan to kick-start your business, I struggle to believe we're the same people. The sleepless nights and endless, hardworking days. We needn't have worried. It was all under control. See how well you've done.

And what made you and Stivvy show your bare arses on the stage in the nightclub? Why the fascination with mooning in those days? Add to that, the countless nights you'd come home from work, half naked, having had your clothes torn off in the pub. And while we're on with nakedness and bare arses, why did you drag me out of bed and chuck me out on the street with not a stitch on? Was it the Becks beer? Booze-soaked terrors?

I felt so proud when you would hunker down, facing the door of any pub or restaurant, sword arm free, ready to defend against potential marauding villains. I am forever safe with you around. Even now.

How vivid are the memories of those nights when no microphone could be left unattended? Long before karaoke burst onto the scene, you would steal the mic from the DJ and lead the audience in animated renditions of songs like *Black Velvet Band* and *Swing Low Sweet Chariot*. I soon knew the words to the lot of them.

How many Saturday afternoons did the house throb with the vibrant strains of your favourite music, which nurtured in our children a deep and everlasting appreciation of Pink Floyd?

And how could I forget those magical mornings when, having stayed up all night, we would grab a couple of flutes and a bottle of champagne, race to the Esplanade to welcome the sunrise with giggles and bubbles, before staggering home to top it all off with scrambled eggs and smoked salmon on toast?

No, Nigel, I won't forget you. I won't forget a single day of the time we've had. MND has stolen our future but it hasn't touched our past. No matter how this disease tries to cloak you in its disguise, the real you will never become invisible to me. Let's remember that.

17

COST MORE THAN OUR FIRST HOUSE

The strident whine of the riser-recliner motor heralds Nigel is on the move.

'Bathroom?'

'Yeah. Sorry to interrupt.'

'Excuse us,' I say, placing my glass on the coffee table. 'Won't be long.'

Not true, we'll be an age. Nothing is achieved in an instant now.

'Shall I wait until you're back?' asks Mel, who holds us engrossed in the drama of an animated tale involving superglue and a lock.

'God no. Carry on.' Don't halt this riveting story. Chances are Mel will sweep us towards the spectacular crescendo before Nigel and I leave the room.

'So, when nobody was around and all was quiet.'

Nigel adjusts the riser recliner to the point where his feet are resting on the floor and his body is leaning forward. I slide the sling across his back and pull the straps under his armpits and beneath his legs. The right way up this time, with a bit of luck. New at this, my manual handling skills are hesitant and clumsy. It looked easy when the Occupational Therapist did it.

'Can we help?' ask Derek and Tom, in unison, worried perhaps by my less than competent performance.

'No don't worry. It's easier with one.' Another untruth. However, two people who don't know what they're doing are twice as abysmal as one.

'So, what happened when the police arrived?'

'Well ....'

Grunting, I manoeuvre the mobile hoist towards what the kids refer to as Dad's control centre. Captain Casson is pleased I ignored his plea to wait until he was dead to refurbish the lounge. He now commands operations from his impeccable post, sited with regimental precision, so all essentials are within reach, and from where he oversees his domain, without the hassle of twisting his head.

'You're joking.'

The riser recliner, flanked by two marble lamp tables bearing the whole shebang of necessities such as man tissues, toothpicks, sweeties, medication, thermostat, fan, and an ever-present cup of tea, is on loan from the MND Association. It is one of the few places where Nigel is comfortable and consequently this is where he spends most of his day.

I do wish it wasn't pink. What is it with pink chairs? Who the hell wants a pink chair?

'And, you won't believe this ....'

Avoiding the clamps gripping the edge of each table, one holding his lap-top, the other, his iPad, and endeavouring not to snag the wheels on the warren of wires stretching like sleeping snakes towards their personal plug point in the den of extensions littering the floor, I manage, at last, to attach the hooks of the sling to the hoist.

'Hurry up, I'm gonna piss meself,' says Nigel, swelling the hilarity already present in the room, Mel's sparkling saga having reached its finale.

I press the button marked with the upward arrow. Slowly, Nigel rises from the chair. The merriment subsides. He hangs, suspended. Dangling like a baby carried by a stork. Defenceless. Exposed. Nobody speaks. Somebody coughs. Someone else sniffs. An uneasy silence descends.

'Does my bum look big in this?' he says.

The brilliant one-liner rips through the tension and riotous laughter erupts into the room.

'Yes, it does, daft bugger,' I say, easing the hoist into position. Good on yer, Nige. Even now, as his condition worsens, he manages to help the rest of us cope.

I lower Nigel into one of the four wheelchairs that form part of the ever-increasing catalogue of care kit occupying space in our home. The collection of chairs all played their part in supporting Nigel through his progressive disability. This one, powered, compact and nippy, ferries Nigel around the place, to and from the wetroom. It was provided by the wheelchair centre, where you might expect the demonstrator to be accustomed to physical disability, and not speak to Nigel as though he was retarded. Nigel's patience as the operational complexities of a joystick were explained to him was astonishing.

Unloved, banished to the gloomiest corner of the garage, covered in cobwebs and buried beneath junk, is the first and last manual wheelchair we ever bought. With confidence borne of ignorance we allowed this abomination of a carriage to accompany us on a long weekend to Brussels. This chair is possessed, compelled by devils to tumble into every pothole, fault and fissure. Or could it be my driving? Being subjected to the incompetence of others, however noble their intentions, is not something Nigel could endure for long and the manual wheelchair had to go. I'm not at all sorry it's exiled.

A sporty, nifty, metallic blue number also resides in the garage. Bought because of its boastful claim to effortlessly climb kerbs. It lied. Nevertheless, it has provided hours of fun as a serious contender in wheelchair races up and down the service road at the back of the house. Despite this, it is now condemned to gather dust with its manual mate.

After significant research, the ultimate in mobile chairs arrives. This gleaming new, top of the range, can-do-anything wheelchair travels for fifteen miles before the battery requires charging. It performs a perfect 360-degree spin on a tanner and tilts and reclines to a sleeping position. Exceptional as it is, further adaptations are necessary to meet Nigel's exacting standards. A made to measure upholstered winged back and headrest are commissioned, along with two additional foam filled seats.

'This cost more than our first house,' he yells, to anyone who will listen, delighted with his customised, original 'Queen Anne' on wheels.

'I'm free!' he shrieks, hurtling down the lane on a mission to buy a paper, as excited as a youngster heading off on a huge adventure.

'Shall I come with you?' I cry after him. He hasn't ventured out alone, for months. Will he manage to pick the paper from the shelf? Will he fit through the shop doorway? If he needs help, will the shop assistants understand a word he says? His response is a joyful wave as the chair rounds the corner and disappears.

The degree of pleasure I know he will derive from this simple jaunt to the shop warms me to my core. What am I saying? He won't settle on a trip to the shop. He may not bother with the shop. If I know Nigel, he will drive the chair up to the top of Oliver's Mount to career down it at speed. Once conquered, he'll test how 'Queen Anne' tackles sharp corners without toppling. He'll drop it off the kerb to monitor its clambering back up efficiency.

I bet he'll head for the path along the golf course and heckle a former combatant to distract him from his stroke.

'Hey, check out this chair mate. Cost more than my first house.'

He'll be reminded of the day he achieved a hole-in-one on the par four, in spite of, or because of, the pounding hangover.

It wouldn't surprise me if he crossed the Spa Bridge into the centre of town. His chair could earn its battle scars by engaging in a joust with those menaces on mobility scooters. He'll barge into stores, toppling tins, crashing crockery and colliding into clothes rails. He might scurry to the skate park on Marine Drive and show the kids some slick tricks as he rides the ramps. He won't mention the cost of his wheelchair to that bunch.

He's bound to bump into old acquaintances and doubtless encounter new ones. He'll laugh and share a joke, tell them his chair cost more than his first house, and add them to his ever-increasing circle of Facebook friends. If he happens upon a gang of scaffolders erecting or dismantling a scaffold, he'll stop and ask if they need a hand. Chances are they will know him because they will have worked for him at some point. He'll let them know what they're doing wrong and invite them to admire his cost-more-than-my-first-house wheelchair.

In the end, MND will take Nigel's life, but it will never lure the joy from his heart, nor dispel the spirit from his soul.

18
STARTING TO DIE

Tap. Tap. Tap.

You're back. I'd forgotten about you. Thought we'd left you in Spain. How stupid. What made you show up again? We don't want you here. We're settled now. In a routine. Lots of procedures. We're in control of this new life and know exactly what to do. We're adapting, managing and learning. We're happy. All the kit, whatever we need, is at our disposal. We don't need you interfering now. You'll spoil everything. Go away. Please. Sod off.

Ah, you're staying right here aren't you? Look at you, spewing your scorn, drumming those disgusting, withered fingers. Tap. Tap. Tapping. Watching. Waiting. Are you enjoying this? Must you smirk?

Don't you dare touch him. Don't lay that putrid hand on his sleeping face. Haven't you finished yet? What more do you want? What is it? You out of practice? Is that the problem? Bored maybe? A soupçon more unspeakable suffering do the trick, will it? Fancy finding new ways of inflicting a tad more torture? I mean, bloody hell, he hasn't complained yet. Not once. You'll need a shitload more creativity to gratify your sadistic desires, mate.

Let's consider your progress, eh? You've destroyed his body. Tick. Devoured the last morsel of his strength. Tick. Shattered the smallest splinter of hope. Job done. So, now what? What's stuffed up your stinking ragged sleeve? Sucking his spirit out through his eyeballs? That do you? Or maybe you could trample all over his soul until he's nothing but a hollow, snivelling carcass? Satisfied?

Well, you won't be doing any of that. I won't let you. Neither will he. So, fuck off.

...

The unremarkable façade of the Leeds St James' hospital, referred to by the locals as 'Jimmy's,' looms unexpectedly from a maze of indistinguishable terraced streets. Pulling into the car park, I defer, grudgingly, to the sat nav. It was right after all. I had envisaged a grander approach and a more imposing exterior for such a famous institution. Ah well, don't judge a book and all that.

We arrive at the respiratory unit early, prepared for a wait. The letter had said to allow three hours for the appointment. As we approach the waiting area, the unwelcome blare of the television greets us. Not this programme please. Nigel manoeuvres into place at the end of a row of seats, while I take one of the mandatory green hospital chairs beside him and try not to gawp at the TV. Not sure how long I can tolerate the insufferable Jeremy Kyle, sermonising with the pompous exasperation of the intrinsically virtuous, as he belittles those hapless, tracksuit wearing, one brain cell apiece cretins, who would willingly part with a kidney for five minutes of fame.

Yet another hospital. Ignoring the television, I count the hours spent in such surroundings. Pink and green, as usual, a splash of baby blue detracting not at all from the array of impractical, insipid colours. All those trips to Sheffield for the lithium trial. No impact. No progress. Still no sign of a cure. And Nigel never did make it to the end of the trial on his feet.

As a rant regarding somebody's boyfriend, accused of scoffing her mother's labradoodle gets underway, Nigel's name is called and we are led to freedom by a young nurse, with a blonde pixie cut and ruddy cheeks.

'Hiya, I'm Leanne,' she says, her West Yorkshire accent evoking memories of my youth. 'We'll do a few tests before you see the doctor.'

'Where're you from?' asks Nigel, would you believe? Although I suspect he, like me, has already guessed. The distinction between the twang of neighbouring towns such as Bradford, Halifax and Huddersfield are significant and instantly recognisable.

''alifax,' she chirrups.

'My hometown,' I say.

'Thought so,' says Nigel. 'You can guarantee a great night out in Halifax. Always end up battling with the bouncers though. Especially in Clarence's.'

'Yeah? That shut down yonks since,' says Leanne.

'I'm not surprised. This particular night, me and our kid –' He stops, chuckling at the memory. 'Our kid gets belted by, oh, no.' He stops again, chokes on a giggle. Here we go, full on elephant trumpeting next. A sure sign he's losing it.

'Spit it out,' she says. 'I'm dying to know what happened.'

Nigel rallies and blurts, 'By a bloke dressed as –' before irrepressible cackling overpowers his story-telling capacity.

'We won't hear the rest,' I explain, resisting the temptation to slap him round the head. 'He'll be a while yet.'

'Must be right funny.'

Leanne attaches a small peg-like device to Nigel's ear. 'You've driven from Scarborough?'

'Yes,' I respond, on his behalf.

'I love Scarborough,' she enthuses, 'I have some patients there. Visit every couple of months.'

'Really?'

'Yes. What's the name of that park?'

'Peasholm?'

'That's it.' Placing her hand on Nigel's quivering shoulder, she adds, 'Now you, I need to hook you up to this machine. Can you stop laughing your head off for a minute?'

Nigel signals his acquiescence by raising his hand and composes himself enough to apologise, 'I'm on drugs,' he jokes. 'I can't help it.' Resting his head, he takes a deep breath and closes his eyes, a wide grin still planted on his face.

'Are you always like this?' asks Leanne.

'I try to be,' he says.

At last, connected and required to do nothing more than breathe in and out for a couple of minutes, Leanne instructs him to blow, as hard as he can, into the spirometer: medical apparatus, she informs us, for measuring aspects of breathing quality.

'All done,' she says, at last, Nigel having accomplished super-human self-control for a massive five minutes. 'Well, that was fun. I wondered if we'd make it for a while there. Wish they were all like you.'

As we head back to the waiting room, she adds, 'Finish that story when I'm next in Scarborough. I'll add you to my list.'

'Look forward to it,' he says, already halfway down the corridor.

Preoccupied by the despicable doggy drama facing Mr Kyle, I give little thought to the prospect of Leanne, yet another medical professional visiting our home. Oh wonderful, he's buggered off. *Heir Hunters*, it is. Could be worse. Before I become engrossed by the government coffers claiming Gladys Ethelberg's fortune, Leanne reappears to deliver us to Doctor Edwards. Happily, cousin Cyril is discovered as we vacate the waiting area.

Compared to Doctor Edwards, Leanne appears sullen. He draws us into his minuscule office with the exuberance of an estate agent flogging a mansion.

'Hello, hello! Grand to meet you,' he booms, his voice in sync with his bulk. He grasps Nigel's hand and shakes it with gusto. 'Do come in.'

In the time it takes for us to wedge ourselves into the cramped space, we indulge in some inconsequential chatter, bemoan the weather, berate the traffic, declare we found the place without difficulty, despite doubting the sat nav, and decline the unusual offer of a cuppa.

'I must say you look exceptionally well,' thunders the doctor, having somehow squeezed his mass behind a desk littered with stacks of papers, haphazard files, three empty mugs and an in-tray resembling a waste-paper bin.

Bet his secretary loves him, I ponder, slipping into my allotted seat.

'I know I do. I am well. Apart from MND.'

Doctor Edwards has no difficulty understanding Nigel's speech, and responds without delay. 'Of course. Which is why you're here.' He glares at Nigel through tortoiseshell framed glasses. 'You're suffering from headaches, I understand?'

'Yes,' starts Nigel and stops short, drained from memories of his antics in Halifax. He shoots me a weary glance to continue to speak on his behalf.

'He's not sleeping well, which is not like him. Waking in the night distressed and panicky. In the mornings he has a nagging headache. Paracetamol doesn't help and the headaches linger all morning.'

'I see. Well, the test results are here and, as I suspected,' he says, waving a piece of paper, 'the outcomes are abnormal.'

'Abnormal?' echoes Nigel.

'Yes,' he continues, in the detached manner of a biology teacher explaining the process of photosynthesis to a pair of twelve-year-olds. 'The disease is now affecting your breathing muscles. It's a common occurrence. Inevitable, in fact. Your carbon dioxide levels are askew.'

We absorb the gravity of this news quietly. I lay my hand on Nigel's arm.

'All over the place,' the doctor continues.

Yes, we know what askew means.

'Right,' says Nigel.

'Hence the headaches.'

'I see,' says Nigel.

'And the panic attacks.'

Doctor Edwards shifts his weight onto his forearms, scattering the papers on his desk and knocking over a mug, which he ignores. An image of a demented secretary aiming a gun at his chest pops into my head. He clasps his paws, purses generous lips and scrutinises Nigel with microscopic intensity.

'Surprised?'

'Yes.'

'Indeed,' he says. 'People expect breathlessness to be the main sign of respiratory problems. In fact, headaches and sensations of panic are classic symptoms.'

Nigel's earlier merriment has now dissolved and he merely nods.

'But look at you!' he bellows, bounding from his desk like a charging grizzly. I uncross my legs and hastily tuck them out of his way under my seat, scrunching up my body to reduce its size, the way I do when I overtake a lorry on a motorway. It's about as effective. Doctor Edwards advances on Nigel and thumps him on the shoulder. 'You're doing brilliantly. For someone with MND you're unusually strong. My God, I wouldn't bet on my chances in an arm wrestle with you.'

We chortle a little. Like you do. I hitch my chair a notch further back.

'We can help with your breathing. We'll set you up with a non-invasive ventilator, affectionately known as a NIPPY, which I suggest you start using for a few hours overnight, increasing an hour each week.'

He might as well be speaking Russian.

'NIPPY?'

'Don't worry, we'll make sure you receive the training before you leave and you should take it home with you today.'

The three-hour appointment now makes sense. Doctor Edwards rests his sizeable rump on the edge of the desk, toppling the in-tray as he does so. That poor bloody secretary. He folds his arms and adopts, what I suppose, is, for him, a rare, sombre expression.

'Now, I must mention, not everybody is comfortable with the NIPPY. You'll need to familiarise yourselves with it. I promise, if you persevere, it will prolong your life. If you don't, it won't. And your life will be shorter.'

I imagine professional disconnection from patients is a training requirement for doctors. How to remain aloof when confronted with a dying person. Calm and precise presentation of the facts, leave no opportunity for confusion, then propose treatment. If there is any.

'How will I die?' says Nigel, from nowhere.

'Sorry?' says the doctor. 'What do you mean?'

Nigel takes a moment before adding, 'I'm worried about choking.'

How did I miss this? I had no idea. Nigel, how long has the manner of your death tormented you? I reach for him, placing my hand on his, by way of apology. As if the action could in any way make up for my ineptitude.

'My fine fellow,' bellows Doctor Edwards, spreading his arms wide as if to embrace and carry us, with the confidence of one who has all the answers, along the road to enlightenment. 'MND results in some magnificent deaths. Magnificent! Not one MND sufferer I know has ever died from choking. Let me reassure you. It won't happen like that.'

'How then?' asks Nigel with unusual insistence.

'Failure of the breathing muscles,' he continues apace. 'However, many deaths result from a chest infection such as pneumonia. Let me assure you these deaths are peaceful and controlled. We know what to expect and when, we are never taken by surprise. I must stress Mr Casson, in many ways, you are a lucky man.'

I raise my eyebrows a touch.

'For example,' he continues. 'There will be some amongst your family and friends, perhaps more than one or two, who are worrying about you, who may well die before you. They are unaware of their imminent death. You, on the other hand, can prepare. Make provision. Say farewell to your family. This is denied so many.

Well, when you explain it like that.

'And, furthermore, you know your death will be painless. We make sure of it.'

'You make sure of it?'

'Yes. When the time comes, we will ensure your comfort.'

'How?'

Doctor Edwards responds without hesitation.

'Morphine. Whatever you need. You will not suffer.'

Nigel takes a deep breath and relaxes into his chair. 'Thank you,' he says. 'I'm OK with the idea of dying, I didn't know how it would actually end. Thanks again, I'm a lot happier.'

'You're welcome,' he beams. 'Now, off you pop and collect your NIPPY. And be sure to persevere. It's your friend.'

...

Our new friend is on the table next to Nigel's bed, occupying the space where the wardrobes once stood. The tubes are attached, the 'breathe in,' 'wait,' 'breathe out' settings, all fixed by our trainer, to alleviate Nigel's current breathing problems. All that remains is to place the headpiece over Nigel's head, make sure the nose pillow, cute name, is the right way up, and switch on the machine. Simple. No, machine on first, headpiece next. Perhaps I should check the instruction manual again?

Later that night, I hoist my exhausted husband into bed, lower him onto the mattress, fold the duvet around him, plump up his pillow and lift the cot sides. Everything is in place and within his reach: iPad clamped on the rail facilitating the entertainment of his many Facebook friends; water, should he be thirsty; extra tablets if he's suffering during the night; sweets should he fancy a treat; tissues to capture the odd sneeze and the alarm, should the impossible occur and I don't hear him call. Only the NIPPY left.

I switch it on and move to fit the headpiece over his face. Nigel grasps my hand and stops me. His tentative smile fails to flush the sorrow from his tired and watery eyes. 'I'm starting to die,' he says. 'Breathing. It's a big deal.'

'I know,' I whisper.

I lay a tender kiss on his forehead. And, as I do, the ghoul at the end of the bed slowly grins.

Tap. Tap. Tap.

19
22 JULY 2011

'Girls! Come on, you must eat. That champagne needs soaking up.'

I plonk the platters of tuna mayo, cheese and onion and ham and mustard sandwiches, cut into triangles and displayed around a mound of crisps, like I cared, on the kitchen island, and dump the Sainsbury wrappers in the bin.

Becky wanders in, clad in bright pink vest and shorts, face half made up and hair still soaked from the shower.

'I'm too nervous to eat.' She refills her flute with the last of the decent champagne. Four bottles of cheap fizz remain on the worktop.

'Force yourself. And take it easy.'

She takes a long sip of the bubbles. 'Don't worry. The bride never gets pissed at her own wedding.'

'Until today, maybe?'

Ellie, make-up bag stuffed under one arm, magnifying mirror in her armpit, grabs a seat, tips the contents of the bag over the island, selects a fine brush and smoky grey shadow and peers into the mirror while reaching for a sandwich. 'You make these?'

'Did I hell. We've a wedding on. Who has time?'

'Is there butter in them?' asks Natalie, her gorgeous face alight with anticipation.

How many times must my niece remind me she doesn't eat butter? 'Oh Nat, I'm so sorry. Shall I stick a pizza in the oven?'

'No, it's alright,' she says, 'I'll make do with crisps and champagne, same as Becky.'

'Girlies,' shrieks Rachel, dashing in. 'Who's next for the hairdresser? I'm all done.' She pats her chin length auburn hair. 'Is that tuna? I don't eat tuna.'

'Cheese or ham perhaps?' I say. 'Or a crisp.'

'You go Nat,' says Becky. 'Ellie, will you finish my face?'

Michele, as pale as death, shuffles in and groans, 'Can anybody do anything with this face?'

'Bloody hell, girl, you look rough,' says Rachel.

I offer the platter. 'Sandwich?'

'Ugh, no thanks,' she gulps. 'I feel like shit.'

'Well, I did scrape you off the bathroom floor at 4.00 am.' I chasten, like I've never sunk so low.

'Was that you? Sorry.'

'Don't be, I'm only kidding. Will somebody please eat a bloody sandwich?'

'Here,' says Becky, placing a flute of fizz in Michele's hand. 'Chuck that down yer neck.'

'Joooleee,' calls Nigel from the bedroom, abandoned there since I showered him at dawn.

'I need to dress your dad. God, there's loads to do. Our Nige will be here in a minute to take photos and look at the state of you lot. And where the hell is Craig?'

'Joooleee.'

'Coming Nig.'

'Mum, breathe,' says Ellie.

'Mum, drink,' says Becky, handing me a flute.

I take a deep breath and down the bubbles in one.

'Right. Get a move on while I sort your dad.'

Please, please don't let the day fall apart before it's started, I beg. I could be an event planner for royalty if the meticulous preparation devoted to this wedding pays off. State banquet? Piece of piss. I wish Nigel had taken Karen's advice and started taking Citalopram. It would be established in his system now. He'd be calmer. Fewer panic attacks. No Girl Guide persuasion badge for you on this occasion, Karen. Of all the nuggets of advice to ignore. 'Worried about becoming addicted,' he said. So what if he does? What does it matter?

The tranquil bedroom soothes like silk the instant I step inside and the air is laced with the potent scent of Becky's exquisite bridal bouquet, laid out of harm's way on my bed. Delphiniums, sparkling like sapphires in a festoon of white trumpet lilies. Stunning. My complementary corsage bracelet and lily buttonholes for the men rest alongside. Did I include Ben and Tom in the buttonhole order? A cursory calculation confirms I did.

Nigel grins at me from his profiling bed, operating the controls to raise himself up. 'How's it going?'

'Bloody madness, as ever.'

'It'll be fine,' he says. Get me dressed and then deal with everything else, without fretting over me.'

'Come on, your suit's all ready.'

This will be fun. I cast a concerned eye over the dapper dove grey jacket and trousers, the double-cuff Savile Row shirt, silver and cobalt blue silk tie and handkerchief. Quite a change from the pull-on casual loungewear. I'll need to dangle him from the hoist to slip his trousers on and zip them up. God knows what we'll do if he needs the toilet at the reception. Whilst the Crown Spa Hotel boasts disabled facilities, there is always the assumption the disabled person is able to transfer in and out of their wheelchair unaccompanied. Not so. Craig and Danny will need to help him. Julie, this is a wedding. Please stop contemplating toilet issues.

'Well Nig, little Becky getting married. Can you believe it?'

'Thought she'd never do it. I'll tell her she's to stay married at least five years or I want my money back.'

'What are you like?' I pant, hoisting him from the bed. 'She will. He's perfect, is Daz. Trousers first?'

'Yeah, OK. Leave the jacket and tie off for now.'

As we perform the complex and unfamiliar mission of coaxing Nigel's body into a suit, my thoughts shift to Becky's soon to be husband. Sergeant Darryl Beattie, loadmaster crewman on Chinook helicopters, attached to No. 27 Squadron, RAF Odiham. No stranger to war zones, Daz has carried out numerous operations involving trooping, supplying and casualty evacuation in Afghanistan and Iraq.

'Another military wedding, Nig,' I say, images of Airforce blue uniforms filling my mind. The striking cobalt of the bridesmaids' gowns will harmonise like a dream. The gymnastics demanded by prizing Nigel's shirt onto his body leaves him breathless, and he blinks his response.

'Which cufflinks?'

'Golf balls.'

We are interrupted by Eleanor's shout. 'Mum. Danny and the boys are here. Is it OK if Danny irons his shirt?'

Why not? It's not as if there's enough chaos. Perhaps I should strip a couple of beds, fill a washer load and maybe run a mop over the kitchen floor?

'Of course.'

'You carry on,' says Nigel, wheeling away from the asylum into the lounge. 'Send Becky in when she's ready.'

Ben and Tom demolish the sandwiches while Danny attacks the creases in his army dress shirt.

'How's the new school?' I ask the munching boys.

Ben grimaces his distaste while Tom rewards me with, 'S'alright, I s'pose.' Having applied and been granted a posting at Catterick so Ellie could be closer to home, Danny, Ellie and the boys now live at Linton-on-Ouse, near York. The RAF treated Becky's application for a northern posting with similar levels of understanding and magnanimity, and she now commutes to RAF Leeming from her married quarters, located on the very next street to her sister. Worrying. I predict mayhem.

'You could eat your dinner off that Jag,' announces Craig, our chauffeur for the day, as he bursts into the kitchen. 'I've got through a full tin of polish. It's shinier than Dad's head. Come and have a skeg before a seagull shits on it.'

'Sorry, I've to don my outfit. Better hope the seagulls are busy elsewhere.'

'Ok, I'll mess about attaching the ribbon to the bonnet, if anybody cares,' he says, departing. He crashes into Nige, who has elected to arrive well in advance of the emergence of the, not so blushing, drop dead gorgeous, bride and bridesmaids yet to erase the hangover shadows from their faces. The bride's mother still to remove these sodding jim-jams and Danny still required to restore the iron and board to the pantry. Not a solitary lily has taken its place in a jacket's buttonhole, a couple of unloved sandwiches continue to dry and curl yet, weird I know, the plonk has vanished.

'Ey up Uncle Nige. Alright?'

'Hi Craig. OK mate?' He places his camera amongst the debris on the island and shakes Craig's hand, then Danny's. 'Greetings, Danny. Bit smart there.'

'Cheers,' says Danny, adjusting the black bow tie of his dress uniform.

Nige, a professional photographer, is far more comfortable capturing images of concrete than people. He's not a fan of wedding photography at all. That being said, our persistent bullying proved stronger than his reluctance, and here he is.

'OJ,' he says, addressing me in his customary way: OJ, short for 'Our Ju'. 'What do you want me to do?'

We've discussed this a million times already. Where's my drink? Deep breath. Breathe. And again. I take the list of must-have shots from my bag and shove it in his hand.

'Here,' I say. 'Do whatever you like, starting now. Please make sure you nail numbers one and two on the list, or I swear I will kill you.'

He glances at the paper before slipping it in the inside pocket of his jacket, where I suspect it will remain for years until he next wears this suit.

'Will do.'

I can only hope. There's no more to be done. Determined to flee the madness and squeeze into my Ian Stuart mother of the bride outfit. I drop the designer's name at every opportunity, like he's a personal friend, and gasp, 'you must have heard of him?' when in reality, it's my way of justifying the expense. At that point, the

vision of my stunning daughter, floating along the hallway, banishes all thoughts of Ian Stuart from my mind.

Elegant folds of delicate fabric caress Becky's petite form as
they flow from a simple fitted bodice. Straps embellished with
pearls complement the subtle headband and dual pearl droplet
earrings, borrowed from Paula. Luxuriant tresses, gleaming and
sensuous as melted chocolate, cascade over one shoulder and her
enchanting oval face, sparkling with happiness, glows beneath her
fringe. She is the epitome of understated grace and sophistication.

'Wow. Look at you.'

'Fabulous, isn't she?' says Ellie, leading the trio of bridesmaids.
Nige grabs his camera and gets to work.

'Is Dad in the lounge? Is he ready?' says Becky.

'Oh yes. Ready and waiting for his moment with his baby. Nige,
you could shoot the bridesmaids, not literally, now they don't look
like they've just been dug up.'

'Don't mess up your eye makeup Bex,' says Ellie, unshed tears
threatening to ruin her own exquiste greasepaint.

Dazzling in their cobalt blue gowns, exhibiting necklines as
daring as Becky's is modest, the girls pose for the camera as Becky
joins Nigel for those precious personal minutes between father
and bride. This is when the proud father, the single most important man in his daughter's life to date, savours his final seconds as
he prepares to hand her to another.

Swallowing the lump in my throat, I rush to the bedroom for
my date with Ian Stuart.

...

The Consort Suite at Scarborough's Crown Hotel buzzes with the
excited murmuring of a hundred-plus guests, already an hour into

the booze. I make my way down the aisle, each row flanked by a tall, floor-standing vase, bearing a single white lily. I take my seat at the front and exchange a wave with my soon to be son-in-law, magnificent in his military uniform, emblazoned with medals and sporting the buttonhole which he attached to the jacket with reluctance, as he suspected the wearing of such adornments was against protocol. Perhaps a military reprimand is preferable to mother-in-law's wrath. Nige, camera poised, is to the right of the Registrar's table. The Registrar checks her wristwatch. Checks it again. It's OK. We're not late. Miracle upon miracle.

The jaunty melody of Israel's *Somewhere Over the Rainbow* trips into the room, along with the swish of swivelling guests eager for their first view of the bride. Gasps of surprised delight and cries of 'Ah wow!' and 'Fantastic!' erupt as Nigel and Becky burst from behind the screen. Becky, her face brimming with joy, is seated upon her dad's knee. Nigel propels his wheelchair down the aisle towards her betrothed, like it's a gilded chariot bearing a princess. Playing to the crowd, he performs a perfect 360-degree spin before crashing to a halt. As Becky alights from his knee, the room thunders with spontaneous applause.

Number one item on the must-have photograph list had better be in the bag, brother Nige.

Here's hoping number two transpires in similar fashion.

...

'Should I usher people outside? In case they're early?'

'They won't be early,' says Daz.

'What if they're late?'

'They won't be late.'

'Oh.'

'They'll be exactly on time, Julie. That's the point.'

All the guests and one or two curious staff are assembled outside the Crown Spa Hotel on Scarborough's Esplanade, overlooking the spectacular south bay. Becky and Darryl, the delightful backdrop of the old town, harbour and castle behind them, pose for photographs. Champagne flutes are filled and filled again. The animated chattering of reunited family and friends shrills like birdsong around us.

'I loved your entrance,' I say, stealing a kiss from Nigel. 'Brilliant idea of Paula's to carry Becky on your knee. Only you could perform it with such panache.'

'Cheers,' he says, offering up his glass. 'It's going well, isn't it?'

'Fabulously. And you, my darling, are remarkable.' As we clink glasses, we hear it.

Wokka wokka wokka wokka wokka wokka.

One hundred pairs of eyes gaze at the headland as the distant thrumming builds to a reverberating beat and, at precisely 1605, the spectacular hulk of a twin-rotor Chinook helicopter bursts into view. The mighty aircraft, like a colossal bee, thrusts along the bay, until it hovers over the sea right in front of us and, displaying astonishing delicacy for such a giant, performs a bow. The clamorous chopping of the rotor blades muffles the cries of our thrilled guests, flapping their arms enough to spill their drinks as they wave at the two pilots and crew members on board. They are so close we can see their teeth gleaming beneath their headgear. They wave back, one of the crew leaning out of the side of the aircraft to hail the bride and groom. Darryl's colleagues, in practising the task of arriving at a specified point at a specified time, pay tribute to Darryl and Becky on their wedding day and honour the rest of us with a unique and unforgettable experience.

Nige, who has observed this marvellous spectacle through his camera lens, continues shooting long after the Chinook has disappeared. The collage of photographs he has scooped is already forming in my mind. It will be placed on the wall alongside Ellie's and Craig's wedding montages. And Nigel will be on it.

'What a wonderful day this is,' I say.

'It is,' says Nigel, draining the dregs of his champagne.

'And do you know why today is so marvellous?' I whisper, leaning close to his face.

'Why?'

'Because you're here. You made it.'

20
EVERY DAY IS A BONUS

The tenth of February 2012 dawns like any other February day. The mournful wail from the lighthouse foghorn soaks into the damp swirling sea-fret shrouding the coastline. The gulls abandon rooftops and chimney stacks, shrieking like tormented souls lost in the mist. Leaden skies deny the feeble winter sun's tremulous light and the raw, piercing cold banishes its warmth.

But not for us. For us, the sun blazes in a sky adorned with fluttering birds, their orchestra filling the air with melodies of sweet, trilling birdsong. Processions of marching bands escort troupes of acrobats and joyful exotic dancers through streets decorated with flags and vibrant bunting. A kaleidoscope of one thousand, eight hundred and twenty-five balloons of every colour float like dazzling butterflies in the wind, each one representing a single day Nigel has stayed alive, since diagnosis.

I place his morning cuppa on the table beside him. He reaches for it with a trembling hand. His movements, now, are slow and hesitant and, like a toddler attempting to pick a solitary crimson button from a mass of green ones, demand concentration.

'My hands are asleep,' he says.

I take the disposable lidded cup and place it in the palm of one hand, curling the fingers of his other, around it. 'Never mind, you've no knitting to finish.'

'Nice one,' he sniggers, before raising the straw to his lips, to sip the sweet, milky tea.

'Five years,' I say. 'Congratulations. You're still here.'

'Yes,' he says, his face aglow. 'Every day's a bonus now.'

Perhaps it is restricted to the terminally ill to truly appreciate the gift of each new day. Many of us breeze through life without recognising the value of anything. Nigel and I, as guilty as any other, spent our working lives in pursuit of wealth and our idea of happiness. Nowadays though, trivial things, like his socks on right, his T-shirt smooth across his back, not too much toothpaste on his brush, are the primary elements of his contentment.

'And we'll treasure them all.' I declare, planting a kiss on his bald head.

'We must,' he says. 'Things could be a lot worse.'

'You're awesome, you know that?' I say, humbled. 'How do you stay so optimistic?'

'Easy. Focus on what I can do, not what I can't.'

'Simple as that?'

'Yes. Try it.'

Taking the empty cup from his outstretched hand I promise to do precisely that. 'Ready?'

Nigel rests his head on the pillow and closes his eyes. Awake ten minutes and already exhausted. 'Give me half an hour.'

'Ok, half an hour. No more.' I tuck the duvet around him. 'Craig's calling for a bacon butty later.' Nigel's already asleep.

Let's have a stab at it, why don't we? This positivity. What is he
still capable of? Top of the list? He thinks. His personality, sense
of humour, hysteria at his corny jokes, remain intact. He still has
the substantial five: touch, sight, hearing, smell, taste. MND will
never steal his senses or mental capacity. No, that's not its style.
MND prefers to ravage the body until it becomes the coffin of the
unchanged person trapped inside. It is beyond cruel.

I'm not doing all that well am I? Come on. Work harder.

Physically, Nigel can breathe, supported overnight by a ventilator, unlike so many sufferers of this dreadful disease who are
unable to breathe at all, without constant help. Yes, this is undeni-
ably something for which we are grateful.

I'm improving. He swallows, holds his cup in both hands and
enjoys the occasional bottle of beer. Sometimes a whisky. Worth a
lot. Especially the whisky. Communicating is gruelling and lacking
in clarity, yet he somehow manages to make himself understood.
Always the determined bugger.

He controls his wheelchair, recliner chair and profiling bed,
choosing to move left or right, sit up, lie back. These are precious
choices. Only when we lose them do we understand. Technology
enables him to challenge the actual proportions of his world.
Online poker, chat rooms, connecting with family and friends, real
and virtual, via his iPad and laptop, gives his life purpose. Not to
mention an audience for his atrocious, politically incorrect gags.
Priceless.

There. I'm on a roll now. What else? We could be skint, Nigel
reminds me time and again. We're not. We could live in a dismal,
decrepit town. We don't. We could be without family. We boast a
fabulous family. Parents, brothers, sisters, kids, actually like one
another. Craig calls in daily. We see more of the girls as Ellie and

Danny now live in Scarborough, having moved here when Danny took redundancy from the Army. Becky and Daz own a house on Castlegate in the old town, visiting their Scarborough base on weekends and holidays.

Yes Nig, you're right. Where we are today could be worse. No valid reason to bemoan today when tomorrow will, in fact, be a whole lot shittier. Don't blow it, Julie. You're doing so well.

...

The smoky fumes of sizzling, spitting bacon pervade the kitchen, setting off the smoke alarm.

'Shit.' I switch on the overhead fan before Nigel becomes distraught.

'Craig, open the doors please, so your dad can breathe.'

Craig slides open the patio doors as Nigel wheels his chair close to the gap to draw a lungful of cold, damp air, while I race into the hall and jump up and down waving a tea-towel beneath the screeching alarm.

'Bacon's burning,' says Craig.

Alarm silenced, I grab the grill pan, switch off the hob, slap the bacon between two slices of buttered white bread and thrust it at Craig.

'Hope it's worth it.'

'You not having one, Dad?'

Nigel, gasping for air, shakes his head.

'No. If the smell doesn't kill him the bacon will,' I explain. 'Scratches his throat. He had an egg butty earlier.'

In the time it takes to make pots of tea for Craig and Nigel, and coffee for me, the smoke dissipates and Nigel breathes once more.

'Big day today, Craig,' he says.

'What d'ya mean?'

'Five years and I'm not dead. In spite of your mother trying to choke me a second ago.'

'Five years? Bloody hell.' Craig bites a massive chunk of the sandwich and, mouth full of bread and bacon, mumbles, 'I don't believe you've got it.'

'Why?'

Craig swallows at last, and adopts a droll, mystified expression, the image of Karl Pilkington from the programme *An Idiot Abroad*. 'Well, isn't MND supposed to be a wasting disease?'

'Yes,' I say.

'Look at you, Dad – you're fat.'

Tea splutters from Nigel's mouth as he jerks forward, snorting with laughter. I grab the cup before he spills the lot on his knee.

'Careful. Is it your turn to choke him?'

'Sorry, I don't know what he'll find funny, do I?'

'He finds everything you say funny.'

At which, Nigel chuckles some more.

I take the drink away. 'You're not drinking any more until Craig's buggered off.'

'I'm not fat,' Nigel says. 'My muscles have flobbered to flab, that's all.'

Craig raises his eyebrows and declines to comment, finishing what remains of his sandwich in silence. I dry Nigel's face, dab the tea from the front of his loungewear top, elevate his feet to his preferred height when in his wheelchair, and sit with my coffee in the cosy tan leather chair in the corner of the kitchen.

'How's your day going?' says Nigel.

'Same shit, different day. Just done a doctor's windows up Holbeck. Acute case of arrogantitis.'

'What do you mean?' I ask.

'Symptoms include severe inflammation of the ego, and the need to talk to window cleaners like they're shite.'

'Oh dear.'

'Anyway, I added his neighbour's place to my round. There I am, standing next to my van. "CC Window Cleaning" painted on the side, ladders on top, hip buckets hanging on my belt, 28-litre bucket of soapy water at my feet.'

'And?'

'This woman comes up to me and says, "Are you a window cleaner?"'

I glance at Nigel, who is grinning, but calm. I shoot a warning glance at Craig.

'And what did you say?'

'No, I re-cover snooker tables.'

That's it. Nigel erupts. Convulsed, his head snaps back, his arms propel forward, and his body shudders. His legs jerk upwards, locked in spasm. Snot bubbles from his nose and a penetrating yowl floods from his mouth.

'God,' says Craig, startled. 'What just happened?'

'You just happened. He's gone into one. Laughing too much.'

'What should we do?

'Nothing.'

I jump up and grab the kitchen roll to clean him when it stops. These attacks, whether a reaction to hilarity or anxiety, are always the same. There is nothing anybody can do. No magic tablet, no soothing words, no comforting embrace. We must wait until the shuddering in Nigel's body subsides and he regains control of his breathing. Craig observes the chilling display in uncomfortable silence. His troubled eyes dart from me, to Nigel and back again. He opens his mouth to speak, abandons the action and clenches his teeth. As the minutes pass Nigel's howling fades to a whimper, his quivering right arm stills a little, and he takes control of the chair, raising it first upright, then forwards, head bowed, until he finds the point where his breathing steadies. Once calmed, the spasm in his legs unlock, and he is still once more.

Craig holds his breath and gawps at his dad. What now?

Nigel raises his head, eyes clamped shut beneath a crinkled brow, cheeks glistening with happy tears and a massive grin splitting his face. 'Fuck me, that was funny,' he says, his voice as coarse as a pebbly beach.

Craig expels the breath he's holding captive in a whoosh. 'Bloody hell, I thought you were gonna die.'

'You should be on the bloody stage,' I joke. 'Bugger off back to work before you kill your dad. Who needs MND with you around?'

'I don't mind dying laughing,' says Nigel.

'Tea?' I ask.

'Yes please.'

'Right, I'm off.' Craig leaps from the bar stool and dashes through the door. He pops his head back into the kitchen. 'Sorry,' he says, with a sheepish grin.

'Don't be,' says Nigel. 'See you tomorrow.'

Nigel drinks his tea before reclining his wheelchair to its extent. His head settles on the headrest. His eyes close. He breathes. And sleeps.

21

DON'T LAUGH AT MY COCK

Nigel is groggy with sleep and still drinking his cuppa when I deprive him of his comfortable bed and barge through his morning routine like a buffalo on speed. Showered, shaved, dressed, breakfasted and settled in the riser-recliner before ten o'clock. Done.

'What if we don't like her?' I rant, twitching at the curtains. 'What do we say? "Sorry you're not suitable, no reason, don't like your face?"'

'Let's meet her, eh?' says Nigel, the embodiment of reason.

'OK, OK. But don't say you like her if you don't. It doesn't matter why. She could be boring, crazy, hideous wart on her nose, creepy sneer, weird walk. Anything.'

'So long as she's not fat,' says Nigel.

'Oh no, what if she is? Are you allowed to be fattist?'

'Don't care.'

'Right. Is a bit on the plump side acceptable?' I say, praying for a skinny carer.

'Maybe. But I'll panic if she crowds me.'

Of course, his claustrophobia. Hadn't thought of that. I hasten to the kitchen, more frantic now than a few seconds ago. The not so perplexing task of tea and coffee preparation fails to halt the angst spinning inside my head. Bloody hell, Julie, get a grip. If her breath doesn't stink like a drain, if she is neither drop-dead gorgeous, which would infuriate me, nor hideous, which would infuriate Nigel, if she's caring and competent, what does it matter? Just not fat. Please God, don't let her be fat.

This is so important. Nigel's first ever carer. It's taken six years for Nigel to reach the point where he needs constant help. Now, he mustn't be alone for a minute.

'It will give you a chance to relax and wander round the shops,' said Karen, on one of her 'what should I talk you into this time?' visits. I hate shopping. 'A trip to the supermarket.' Deep joy. 'Visit your hairdresser.' Tempting. The grey is raging. 'Be pampered.' No thanks. My hairdresser doesn't pamper. That's why I like her. 'How about three hours a week?'

We give in. 'OK, three hours a week.'

'To begin with,' adds Karen. 'You don't appreciate how much care you need until you start with it.'

Well, we'll see, missus know it all. Three hours will be plenty.

The ghost of a quality manager lurks within me still, and I check the magnificent training programme for the hundredth time. Arrogant I know, but it's damn good. Some might consider it over the top, however it strikes me as fastidious prep to compile a file which assumes I will die on my first trip to the supermarket, leaving the carer to attend to Nigel for the rest of his life. This A4 presentation book, with forty sheer display pockets, will ensure the carer is adequately supported. All essential aspects of his care are identified by easy-to-read bullet points, along with colour-coded reference material. Yes, it's all there. Medication chart with administration times and doses. Nigel's likes and dislikes. More than a full page for that one. The dos and don'ts in his routine. Another page. How many sugars in his tea. How strong he likes his coffee. The spoon for feeding him breakfast. Indeed, what he eats for breakfast. The myriad of equipment – what it is, where it is, when it's utilised, how it's handled, how it's cleaned, how to –

The doorbell rings. It's her. I approach as though expecting the bailiffs, and open the door a mere crack. Thank fuck. She's skinny as a toothpick and tall as a pylon. The only space she'll fill is vertical. I swing the door wide. Late forties, straight greying hair crumpled into a tortoiseshell claw and an aged, crinkled face, plundered by perpetual hard work.

'Hello, come in. I'm Julie. Pleased to meet you.'

'Hiya,' she croaks, in a forty-a-day voice. 'I'm Alison.'

'Come and meet Nigel.'

'Where're you from?' he says – imagine that – as Alison takes his hand. Delighted to discover she is a fellow Bradfordian, there follows a discussion on which one of them hails from Bradford's roughest area. Nigel, a lad from Buttershaw council estate, rendered infamous back in 1987 by the film *Rita, Sue and Bob Too*, emerges the victor. Next an update on the current no-go zones and a crawl round the pubs and clubs of Nigel's youth.

I drag the discussion back to the interview it's supposed to be. 'What's your experience in this sector, Alison?' Spoken like my expertise in the care sector is infinite.

Eyes the colour of dish water dig into mine. 'A carer for eight years,' she says with assurance. 'Supervising a team for the last five.'

Nigel interrupts and she waits, paying close attention, as he struggles to form the words. 'Have you cared for anybody with MND?'

'No,' she says, 'but I've read up on it. I'm sure we'll cope. Not been beaten yet.'

Her chortle doesn't manage to illuminate a face ingrained with hardship, and I persist with, 'What kind of care did you provide?'

'Complete personal and home care, round the clock.' She takes a tissue from the side pocket of a large black Tote bag and holds it to her nose as she sniffs. On the verge of tears, she tells us of the recent death of her previous charge. A young man left quadriplegic following an accident and unable to communicate as a result of a stroke. She shouldn't struggle with MND.

CV explored, Bradford toured, cup of tea downed, Alison jumps to her feet and declares, 'Right, let's get on with the caring.'

What? Now? No preparation? No discussion? Before my file is even opened? Before the extent of my responsibilities in performing Nigel's routine, painstakingly outlined in the bloody tome, are considered? This is not your bog standard list of stuff to do, to be handed over to anybody, like it's of no consequence. This is my life.

'It's done,' I say, masking my annoyance. 'You know, cleaning up for the cleaner kind of thing.'

'Oh,' says Alison, dissolving into her chair. 'Sorry, I expected to crack on with the job.'

'Start tomorrow,' says Nigel.

So much for a post-interview discussion.

'Great, what's the first task? Out of bed and into the shower?'

'Yes, that's right. Here,' I hand my precious resource to this confident woman as though parting with the Holy Grail. 'Take this home and read it. It covers all you need to know.'

175

'Brilliant, thank you.' To be fair to her, her gratitude does appear genuine and she places the dossier in her bag with respect, although maybe the gentle pat on its side was a tad over the top. Regardless, I've formulated some questions to test she's read it. 'I'll be here tomorrow morning. Seven-thirty sharp.'

'One more thing,' says Nigel, grinning like he's found a discarded tenner in his pocket.

'Yes?'

'Don't laugh at my cock.'

Alison sniggers like a dog clearing its throat, 'Ha! Well, I wouldn't dream of it. But I will now.'

'I like her,' says Nigel, once I've seen her out.

'Yes Nig. That's obvious.'

...

Irritating, wise old Karen is right. It is impossible to cram the range of out of house activity into three short hours and, over a few months, the hours creep upwards until Nigel has care each weekday morning. Donna, a vivacious and attractive young colleague of Alison's, joins the team and, whilst not as proficient as her mentor, is confident enough to defy Nigel's instructions, and hoots with laughter when presented with his cock.

Nigel embraces this latest development with relish. The tedium in his life is now sprinkled with fragments of absorbing discovery. He explores Alison's and Donna's histories, engages with their stimulating stories and delights in the attention he receives when sharing his own sparkling tales, precious memories and appalling jokes.

As for me? My enthusiasm for what I regard as an intrusion is slow to flourish. I am hesitant to take a step back. Reluctant to let go. Others, not me attending to Nigel's personal needs, nags at me. He, however, is loving every minute of it. This also irritates me. Someone else's giggling instead of mine reverberates from his bathroom and I wonder if he's entertained me with that particular story? That one-liner? The carers execute these routine tasks with alarming ease, like it's not remotely difficult, and my forty-page bible gathers dust in the cupboard. Am I fearful of having my nose pushed out? Becoming redundant? Or jealous, perhaps?

There are mornings I'm overjoyed to spend a few hours alone, and will wander round the shops gazing at garments I neither desire nor need. There are also times when there is no conjuring a reason to flee, and I'm like a visitor in my own home. I accept the polite offer of a coffee and try and relax, as another woman fills my kettle, retrieves crockery and coffee from cupboards she knows as well as I, and presents me with the cuppa while she prepares my husband's breakfast and spoons it into his mouth. If all tasks are completed before the shift is over, I am often unable to tolerate chit chatting for the sake of it, and usher the carers out of the door as soon as it doesn't appear rude to do so.

As the months pass I become accustomed to the presence of carers and settle into this new situation. There is no reason to suppose I am to be subjected to anything else. My irrepressible daughters, however, have other ideas.

'Mum, let's surprise Dad with a puppy for his birthday,' says Becky.

'What? Don't be daft.'

We're not doggy people, in fact, I struggle to suppress a yawn when dog lovers regale me with tales of their pooch's personality. On the other hand, Ellie's and Becky's dogs, Pepper and Silva, succeeded in stealing our hearts. To be fair, miniature schnauzers are way too cute to be considered dogs.

'Look at the baby schnoozers,' says Becky, shoving her phone in my face. Two adorable fluffy puppies fill the screen. 'I'm buying one of them to keep Silva company when me and Daz are at work.'

'You can't leave one behind, Mum,' says Ellie.

'They're the last of the litter.'

'I've never hankered after a dog. Looking after your two is different. I can give them back.'

'What about Dad though?'

'Your dad's never wanted a bloody dog either. He wouldn't let Pepper in the house when you first brought her home, remember?'

'True,' says Ellie 'Then he met her, and boom, true love.'

Desperate now. 'Where will I find the time for a dog?'

'What? You've a shitload of carers.'

'Oh yes. Lucky me.'

'Come on, Mum,' pleads Becky. 'It's Dad's birthday.'

'He might not celebrate many more,' whispers Ellie.

That's it. They win. 'You evil bitches.'

'Ha ha. Knew we'd wear you down,' says Ellie, planting a kiss on my cheek.

Becky reaches for her phone to secure the merchandise before they're snapped up. 'Ah thanks Mum. Love you.'

When Becky presents Nigel with a choice between the two brothers, once recovered from the shock, he opts for the tiny, timid one.

'A Disney dog,' he says, bubbling with delight. 'I'll call him Bodger.'

Becky places Bodger on Nigel's knee. 'There you go Bodger, meet your new dad. My baby boy's name is Milo.'

'God help us, what have I done?'

It soon becomes crystal clear. When people say 'dogs are for life,' I didn't realise it was a swap. As in, you get the dog and the dog gets your life. As carers are in situ and therefore there's not a single thing for me to do, it isn't the slightest bit of bother slotting three walks a day into my non-existent schedule. Not to mention accompanying Bodger into the backyard at two in the morning, huddled against the driving rain, tiptoeing amongst the slugs and indulging in a ridiculous display of exuberance once he does his thing. And why would it pose the slightest problem for my once-immaculate home to be littered with puppy paraphernalia, and to double as his toilet? It is also of zero consequence when the supposedly timid Bodger takes on the mantle of devil-dog and tries to murder me with discarded toys, or by launching himself at my frazzled feet.

Within weeks, this tiny bundle weaves his way into our bosom and Nigel and I become the people we once mocked. Here we are, revelling in Bodger's personality as though he is an actual person, convinced he understands whatever we say to him, assured he is the cleverest dog that ever lived and in tune with how grief-stricken we would be if anything should happen to our precious pet. Alison and Donna, both dog owners, respond to this new addition to our gang with their customary efficiency and their knowhow in removing accidents from long-haired rugs is invaluable.

Once we have settled into this new routine, it changes again. Donna announces she's leaving. I half expect her to be off to university as I've nagged her for months to make something more of her young life than working with the dying. As it is, she is leaving to pursue a career supporting troubled teenagers. Not sure which is worse.

Before I worry about her replacement, Ellie sacrifices her job of teaching assistant supervisor at teenage-ridden Pindar School and leaps in to fill the gap. The 'don't laugh at my cock' directive is rewarded with a slight raising of an elegant eyebrow, and Ellie slides into the role of caring for her dad like butter in a skillet. She's another who fails to consider the need to blow the dust from the discarded 'how to care for Nigel' guide.

In the majority of cases, motor neurone disease progresses rapidly and kills within two years of diagnosis. However, Nigel's MND is slow. His proceeds along a path featuring a series of plateaus and pits. We remain on these plateaus for months. They become secure, manageable sanctuaries. Like finding your way around a new town, you tentatively explore its primary arteries, commit certain landmarks to memory and, with each subsequent trip to the shops, vary the route, discover a couple of shortcuts, until you navigate the map of roads, pathways and back alleys with confidence. Soothed by this growing competence, the violent reminder of war comes as a shock, when a missile explodes right in the centre of town, shattering that precious plateau to pieces. Our familiar territory, our safe haven, annihilated in an instant. And there, crushed and mutilated in the depths of the cavernous pit, is Nigel.

He emerges weaker and more disabled. Far worse, his once unconquerable spirit suffers a savage assault, and some of its sparkle begins to seep, unchecked, from this new wound. Launched yet again into an alien world, a new, unexplored, frightening plateau, our ragged emotions, lack of tolerance and short tempers combine to trigger the cry for additional care.

...

'Mrs Casson, may I emphasise how difficult it is to recruit carers?'

Martin Jones, care manager of Living Independently, rests his harried head in one hand and extends the other towards me, palm upwards, pleading for sympathy. I blink at him. Unmoved.

'Especially carers who are, well, slim.'

'Slim isn't necessary,' I say. 'Just not huge.'

'Again,' he thrusts himself back in his chair like I'd pushed him. 'As I say. Difficult.'

Cheeks, having bloomed from pink to purple in the last few minutes, colour an otherwise insipid face. Wisps of grey hair struggle to maintain their hold on a balding head and a lampshade salt and pepper moustache hovers above thin lips, imprisoned so fiercely between his teeth I think he's striving not to cry.

'Mr Jones,' I say, with all the empathy I can summon. 'I understand how difficult this must be. I'm also aware of how politically incorrect this is.'

He clamps his lips tighter than a miser's wallet.

'However, this is about Nigel. He is the one who is terminally ill. Carers need to hold him, lift him, help him move and change position. He is claustrophobic. When he suffers an attack, because he feels smothered, he breaks into a sweat, his entire body shudders and he has difficulty breathing. He has struggled with three carers you've sent us. It's intolerable. This is his life. His money. His rules.'

The care manager surveys me in silence, inhales a long, deep breath and exhales in a whoosh. 'I understand.'

'Are you able to provide us with appropriate carers or not?' Might as well be direct. There are other providers.

'Yes of course,' he says, surprising me with his conviction, as a minute ago he appeared in danger of tearing out what's left of his hair. 'Give me a week.'

...

Now, eight years into MND, an established team of six carers cover twenty-four hours a day. Except for the afternoons. The afternoons are sacred. This is our time, when we're alone as a couple.

Our carers, all female except for Peter, who, it's worth saying, remains underwhelmed when confronted with Nigel's cock, are now friends. We are at ease with one another and confident in Nigel's care, administered with compassion and dignity and with immense good humour. Despite this dreadful disease, laughter looms large in our home. The bulk of our days, however, are grindingly dull and dominated by procedure. The same things are done every single day, in the same way, at the same time. The forty-two sequential steps for settling Nigel into bed are performed with such fluency we could be dancing on *Strictly*. The familiarity of routine becomes its own comfort blanket. It keeps you sane. But there are times, when the interminable, mind-numbing sameness is overwhelming. These are the days when frustration triumphs over patience. On the rarest of occasions, the banality of our existence is enlivened: like the summer of 2014, when we all – including Nigel – joined the Ice Bucket Challenge in raising money for MND, giggling and screaming as buckets of ice cold water were chucked over our heads. Those joyful days, where you can allow yourself to believe you might be making a difference, that you are somehow helping to beat this thing, are scarce. The Ice Bucket Challenge raised an astonishing $220 million worldwide, and the MND Association received over £7 million in just three months.

'Go on that holiday,' urges Nigel, when asked by Paula and Tom if I'd like to join them on a trip to Malta. 'There's no point both of us rotting in jail.'

'I can't leave you,' I say. 'I've never been away without you.' The odd day perhaps, yes, but not for a whole week. I'll never forget that long lunch in York with Ellie and Becky. Alison had said we could stay out for as long as we liked. Nigel was being prepped for bed when we arrived home. Relieved of my bedtime duty for the first time ever, I couldn't stop crying. I felt I'd abandoned him. Also, the night Paula and I attended the performance of Dr Hook, at the Spa. What an entertainer. What a fantastic evening. Until, halfway through 'I Don't Want To Be Alone Tonight', a torrent of grief overwhelmed me and I fled from the theatre and raced home. I sent Alison away, stationed myself by Nigel's bedside, and wept long into the night.

'Yes, you can,' he says. 'You need a break. I'll be fine.'

It's true. He'll be fine. How couldn't he be? His carers are so accomplished I'm pretty much redundant.

'Who will sort out your bollocks?' I say, as the undisputed champion bollock adjuster. When the delicate arrangement of Nigel's genitalia is called for, I will not be toppled from my podium.

'We'll manage.'

'Replaced so easily, am I?'

'OK. I'll wait for you with my balls in a knot. Go.'

'You sure?'

'I'm sure.'

'I'll be worried about your bollocks.'

'Don't be.'

So, I pack my bag in anticipation of a week on the sunny island of Malta.

...

The balcony of our luxurious apartment overlooks the elite complex of Portomaso Marina, close to St Julian's Bay. The serenity of the marina, where the super rich moor their toys, is disturbed only by a single crewman hosing the deck of one of the apparently deserted megayachts. Where are the owners of these pleasure vessels, I wonder? Enjoying a drink in the Vista Lobby of the five-star Hilton hotel, which dominates the port? Perhaps popped along to their incomparable villa, with sun-soaked terrace and infinity pool sunken in exquisite gardens? Or sampling cuisine from around the globe from the array of classy restaurants skirting the marina?

I don't care. My stomach is churning.

'Ready?' says Paula from inside the apartment.

'Yes. Coming.'

Paula and Tom could not be more considerate if they swaddled me in silk, transported me through Malta in a golden chariot and fed me from a silver spoon.

'Where are we heading?'

'We thought we'd show you Paceville,' says Paula. 'It's not far. And we'd rather go during the day, because it's bedlam at night.'

'And we are far, far too old for that night scene,' adds Tom.

'Great,' I say, relishing the freedom from making any decision other than which shorts to don. 'Let's do it.'

I could still be tired from the flight, although I doubt it. It might be the searing Maltese sun, which I also doubt, but the swirling in my belly stops me five hundred metres into the walk.

'I'm going to be sick.'

'Come on. Let's get back,' says Paula.

We flee to the apartment where I lock myself in the bathroom.

'You OK, Julie?'

'Yes, I must have eaten something that didn't agree with me.'

Lie. I've eaten exactly the same as Paula and Tom and Paula knows it.

'Listen, we'll go to the pool and wait for you there,' she says. 'Will you be alright?'

'Yes definitely. You go. I just need a minute.'

I hang over the toilet bowl. Nothing. I stand, bent in half, my head between my knees and take deep, shuddering breaths. Nothing. I sit on the bathroom floor with my legs hugged to my chest. Nothing. I can't shake the nausea. For God's sake, Julie, throw up!

It wasn't my old mate, the grim spectre of Death, that leapt from my case when I opened it: it was guilt. Guilt at leaving Nigel behind. Guilt at the prospect of having a good time without him. Is this how the holiday is to play out? Will it weigh like a brick in my belly all week? Will the image of Nigel, ill, in bed, ever leave my mind? Will I be able to marvel at the view from the apartment and not grieve because he's not with me?

Get a grip. Ring him.

Abandoning the bathroom, I sit on the balcony and Facetime Nigel. Alison's craggy, work-worn face fills the screen.

'He's asleep,' she whispers. 'He's had a bad morning. Maybe better if you ring tonight.'

'Is he OK?'

'He's fine. Sleeping, now.'

I'm dismissed before I can ask why he's had a bad morning? What have you done? What haven't you done? What are you bloody doing? My questions unanswered, I join Paula and Tom at the pool. I'll ring tonight, when it's Ellie's shift. Find out what the hell is going on.

The holiday whizzes by, as holidays do, with leisurely bouts of sunbathing by the Hilton's pools, and obligatory sightseeing. Nigel accompanies us, in my mind, on every trip. We successfully hike to the busy resort of Sliema, and I try to squash my horror as I contemplate the difficulty Nigel would have manoeuvring his wheelchair through the clamouring bars and cafes that crowd the pavements there. I can't help but scour the ferry for the access ramp as we board it to take us across the bay to the capital of Valletta and I stop myself from remarking, as we explore the bustling grid of ancient, narrow streets that, when the Knights of St John built the city, they did not concern themselves with the needs of disabled people.

It's impossible not to marvel at the Barrakka panoramic lifts and I hold my breath as it drops us, in twenty-five terrifying seconds, from the height of Valletta's fortifications to its thriving Waterfront, where we mingle with cruise liner passengers, and enjoy a refreshing gin and tonic.

I smile and pose for pictures and instantly forward them to Nigel. I enthusiastically recount our day's adventures every evening in our Facetime chats, just before we head out for dinner in one of the lavish restaurants around St Julian's Bay, where I submerge the stubborn queasiness with wine.

Before the combination of sun, sights and fine dining has had the opportunity to perform its magic and permit me to relax, it's time to leave.

'How was it?' says Nigel, as I drag my suitcase into the hall and bend to kiss his cheek.

'Lovely, thank you.'

'Feel better?'

'Much. You were right. I needed the break.'

'Good. I'm glad.'

'How are your bollocks?'

'Knotted to fuck. Thank God you're home.'

22
TOILETING MATTERS

Unless we are destined to die young and in perfect health, at some point in our lives the toilet, and all things toileting, will, like an omnipresent god, dominate our existence. If we progress beyond the tell-tale dribble or Tena Lady tinkle and become old and frail, the simple task of reaching the blessed throne on time is elevated to heroic proportions. 'Better not go any further,' when at the thirty feet away point. 'Mustn't be out long, need to hurry back,' after half an hour of a jaunt outdoors. For many of us, far worse than the occasional accident *en route*, is being stripped of the ability to perform our toileting needs in private and unaided. Regardless of the dignity-enhancing wash and dry toilet in Nigel's wetroom, the degree of his disability means his privacy was denied him some time ago.

'I need a piss,' he yells, following a long and harrowing twenty-four hours, when Ellie and I place him on and off the toilet for what must be the hundredth time. 'But I can't go.'

We fasten the sling around him and hoist his trembling body into his wheelchair. His legs are locked in spasm, so rigid an elephant could cling to those shins and fail to buckle the knees. Ellie struggles to force Nigel's non-compliant limbs into place. 'Try and relax, Dad.'

'Am I braying?' he says, unintelligible to most.

'Like a donkey giving birth,' she mutters.

The violent quivering prevents him giggling at the image of a birthing donkey and I place two Lorazepam on his tongue. 'He's in shock. I'm calling the doctor.'

One hour later, Doctor Morgan, a beanpole of a man with a quiet, gentle demeanour, arrives and takes control.

'Hospital,' he says. 'You need a catheter, fast, before there's any damage to your kidneys. I'll call an ambulance.'

'We'll take him,' says Ellie, reaching for the keys of the adapted Berlingo parked outside. 'We'll be there in fifteen minutes.'

'No, an ambulance will be better,' says the doctor. 'I'll arrange one now.'

Part of me agrees with Ellie, we should make our own way. That said, I wouldn't dream of contradicting a doctor. I am, however, prepared to insult him by instructing him in what he should say. 'Make sure they know he's in a wheelchair,' I insist. 'There's no way of transferring him onto a trolley. Make sure they're aware he has MND.' I realise I'm pressing the point. I don't care. When it's to do with Nigel's MND, I know more than any doctor. 'They'll need a ramp at the back of the ambulance. They must understand.'

He hands me a letter for the team in A and E. 'I will, don't worry.'

'Is it OK for me to give him Lorazepam as he needs it?' I ask, squeezing another from its foil casing. 'It calms him.'

'Yes, of course,' he says. 'The ambulance should be here within the hour, but it's not like *Doc Martin* on the telly you know, if it's not a blue light emergency, it's a ball-ache, even when I ring for it.'

'Like I said,' says Ellie, not succeeding in keeping it under her breath. 'We should take him ourselves.'

'No, no, it will be fine,' he says, on his way out of the door.

The *Doc Martin* programme is a mystery to me, although I know reality will disappoint and won't compare with fiction. I'm right. Sixty-eight long minutes later an ambulance arrives.

'Sorry love, nobody told us you needed a wheelchair accessible ambulance.'

'You're kidding, aren't you?'

'No.'

'Well, how long before one comes?'

'Tomorrow, maybe.'

'For fuck sake!' spits Ellie. 'Come, on let's drive ourselves. Like I said in the first place.'

Who should I scream at first? Doctor Morgan? The ambulance crew? The moron who took the call? Every last sodding one of them? No. Calm down. Help Nigel into the Berlingo. Give him another magic blue serenity tablet. Swallow one yourself? Write a scathing letter of complaint tomorrow.

The anaesthetising Lorazepam does what it says on the packet and he trundles along the corridor like a drunk traversing a tightrope on a unicycle. Nurses pin themselves to the wall as he hurtles past. Patients, incapable of dodging out of the way, resign themselves to certain death and stare at the oncoming vehicle, paralysed with fear. Ellie lunges for the controls. She grabs Nigel's hand so fiercely the golf ball atop the joystick flies off and hurtles down the walkway like a bouncing bomb. The chair crashes to a stop, propelling Nigel forward.

'Woaah.'

'Ouch!' barks Ellie, face contorted in pain. 'You're on my foot.'

The golf ball clatters against the far wall, trips into a tea trolley and slides along the skirting before spinning back. The yellow orb captivates all present. I squeeze past Nigel's wheelchair and retrieve the offending sphere from its resting place: an exposed big toe peeping from a plaster cast belonging to a youth with curly ginger hair and smiling, amber eyes.

'Sorry,' I whisper, to anyone listening.

'Ooops,' says Nigel.

I replace the golf ball on the joystick. As Nigel reaches for it, Ellie blocks him. 'Not a chance,' she says. 'I'll take it from here.'

Having inched our way into a cramped treatment room, empty barring a trolley bed and miniature chair, blue for a change, not the tiresome pink or green I associate with hospitals, we are joined by a striking young doctor who could grace the cover of *Vogue*. Her hair is streaked blonde and clamped into one of those non-messy, messy buns other people can achieve. Her skin is smooth, flawless and bronzed. How she had time to study to become a doctor with the demands of her beauty regime is beyond me. And still not a day over eighteen.

'Hello. Mr Casson?' she trills, in a tuneful and distinct European accent. 'I am Candia. I am to take blood and your temperature.'

As she holds a thermometer to his ear, Nigel, driven by his customary mind-boggling compulsion, asks, 'Where are you from?'

Candia's brow puckers. 'Sorry?'

I leap to translate. 'He's asking where you are from?'

'Ah, so sorry.' Perfect white teeth gleam at us as she says. 'I'm from Crete.'

The slow-spreading grin and dancing devil igniting those twinkling eyes should compel me to grab the tourniquet she is placing around his arm and wrap it instead round his neck. I miss my chance.

'A cretin?' he says.

'My God,' whispers Ellie, ramming her knuckles into the arm Candia is not preoccupied with.

'No, a Cretan,' he concludes, emphasising the 'ee' sound.

Ellie eases the pressure a little.

'Sorry?' says Candia again, focused on her third attempt to draw blood from his mean veins and, I'm happy to say, unable to understand a word.

'It's the drugs,' I stutter. 'Affects his speech.' Glaring at Nigel, I shove another Lorazepam in his mouth. We must be up to six now.

'At last,' she heralds triumphantly and extracts sufficient blood to fill the tube. 'We'll test this. However, your temperature is high. We need a chest x-ray to check for infection.'

'What happens if he has an infection?' I ask.

'We will admit him.' She makes to leave. 'My colleague will fit the catheter soon. Goodbye Mr Casson.'

'Bye,' says Nigel, grinning still.

'Thank you,' I say. Admitting him would be a nightmare. How would they cope with him? Hospitals are not equipped for people with MND. And then there's Nigel, and his MND.

'You bloody cretin.' says Ellie, punching Nigel's arm. 'You actual, bloody, cretin.'

'I was only joking.'

'Lucky you stayed in bray mode. You might as well have been speaking Greek.'

'She'd understand that.'

'Ha ha. One more word and I'll kill you.'

'Not if I kill him first,' I add, like a devoted wife.

The door opens before either of us carry out our threats and another child doctor enters. I'm of the age where doctors, teachers and policemen appear young enough to still attend school.

'Mr Casson?'

'Yes.'

The doctor acknowledges me and Ellie with a polite nod. He scrutinises Nigel. 'Hi, I'm Dan, here to make you more comfortable. Does this wheelchair lean back?'

'Yes it does the lot. Cost more than our first house,' says Nigel reclining his chair. 'Where are you from, Doctor Dan?'

Ellie rolls her eyes. The doctor frowns.

'He's asking where you're from,' I translate, choosing to ignore the first house bit. I'm sure the doctor won't care.

'Oh, I see. Nottingham.'

Ellie and I exchange glances. Safer territory this. Still, I hold my breath and wait for Robin Hood to be lobbed into the pot. We're spared. Nigel remains silent as the doctor prepares his equipment. 'This may hurt a bit,' he says. Nigel signals for yet another Lorazepam to help things along. How many of these does it take to overdose?

I daren't watch as Doctor Dan does his stuff and I'm grateful when, a few short minutes later, Nigel gasps with relief as a stream of golden urine gushes unchecked into the waiting bag.

'You've blinded my one-eyed snake.'

'He says he feels a lot better, thank you,' I say, while Ellie once again grinds her knuckles deep into his flesh.

'Excellent. Someone will be along to show you how to change the bag,' he says, departing. 'Best of luck, Mr Casson.'

Nigel is close to sleep. Perhaps exhausted by the stress of the morning, or more accurately, paralysed by Lorazepam. When, an hour later, we are summoned to x-ray, he is still drunk with fatigue. He jerks his chair along the corridor like a chimp let loose on a dodgem, snagging the tube protruding from that hypersensitive part of his anatomy and dragging it beneath the wheels.

'Ow!' he yells. 'That hurt.'

'Slow down, Nig. Steady on.'

I grab the bag of urine and hold it and the tube as far away from him and the chair as is possible without inflicting yet more pain. Ellie crabwalks in advance of us, determined to save her bruised and swollen foot from those treacherous wheels. The x-ray proceeds without drama and we make it back to our treatment room to await the results, unharmed.

'I need the toilet,' says Nigel, after five minutes.

My eyes flit from his face, to the catheter bag and back again. Has he forgotten the catheter?

'You sure?'

'I'm sure. There's no bag for this.'

'Ah, of course. Sorry. Leave it with me.'

I slip out in search of a nurse. There must be a disabled facility with a ceiling hoist.

This is a hospital. Bound to be. How could there not be? We've brought the sling. We're prepared. This won't be a problem. It's a problem. No such toilet facility.

'What? You're joking? OK. A commode? You must possess one of those? And a mobile hoist please.'

I race to our cell and open the door to find Nigel pressed hard against the back of his chair. His eyes screwed shut. The noise coming from him has advanced from birthing donkey to distressed elephant. His hands quiver and his legs are once again locked in spasm.

'I've given Dad another tablet,' says Ellie, her aqua green eyes swamped with anxiety. 'He's gone into one.'

'OK, don't worry.' I cool his soaking brow with a wet wipe, one of the many 'in case we need it' items we throw in the bag when we leave home. Not unlike caring for an infant. Except this infant weighs thirteen stone. 'Won't be long Nig. Hang in there darling.'

A nurse enters the room wheeling a commode.

'Here you are,' she enthuses. 'Can you manage?'

Yes sure. This levitation lark is a piece of piss. Couple of magic words and up he floats. Abra-ca-bloody-dabra. Sha-sodding-zam. 'Would you have a hoist by any chance?'

'Oh.' She takes in the scene. A shuddering, trumpeting man in a wheelchair flanked by two frazzled women, one young, strong and battle ready, the other, menopausal. Both at the point of losing their sanity. She flushes like she's stumbled into a radioactive zone without her HazMat suit. 'I'll send one from the ward.'

'It could well be too late.' I hiss through gritted teeth, Nigel's increasing distress transmiting like prickly heat.

Two nurses arrive at last. They struggle with the hoist like they're dragging it through a swimming pool. It is obvious they are as unfamiliar with this piece of kit as *Ab Fab's* Patsy and Eddie would be dishing out tea at an Alcoholics Anonymous meeting. Faces pink with exertion, one shoves at the rear, the other tugs from the front. Ellie holds the door open. They ram the hoist into the doorframe again and again.

'Give it here,' I fume, lifting it from their hands and forcing the contraption into the room.

The hoist, Nigel, his ramrod legs, colossal wheelchair, a commode and four women crammed into a space intended for no more than one doctor and one patient and, at a push, a tiny person occupying the blue chair in the corner.

'We'll manage, now, thanks,' I say, dismissing the nurses.

'You sure?' says Patsy.

'Certain. There's no room as it is,' snaps Ellie.

'What if we leave the door open?' says Eddie.

I gawp at her. Did she actually say that? 'Where's the dignity in that?'

'Sorry,' she says.

'Leave, please.'

At last, the door closes behind them.

'Were we rude?' I say.

'A bit,' says Ellie.

'Do we care?'

'No.'

'Sorry. No way would Patsy and Eddie have a hope of dealing with your poor dad. Look at the state of him.'

'This won't be easy' she says, taking hold of Nigel's trembling shoulders and leaning him forward. I slip the sling behind him and under his armpits. Ellie attaches the straps to the hoist as I force the leg sections beneath his thighs and hook the straps in place.

'OK,' I say, 'You shift the chair out of the way, while I hoist him.'

'Hurry,' cries Nigel.

'Nearly there, Nig.'

'Ow. My bloody foot,' squeals Ellie.

'Quick.'

The chair slams into the trolley bed. I squeeze the hoist between the bed and the wall and twist while Ellie slips the commode into the gap.

'There you are darling,' I say, when Nigel is settled. 'We'll wait outside.'

Out in the corridor, we lean with our backs against the wall and take long, deep breaths.

'I need a fag,' says Ellie.

'Thought you'd stopped?'

'I have.'

'How's your foot?'

'Throbbing.'

'I'm ready,' calls Nigel.

Dashing back into the treatment room we find him slumped on the commode, head lolling onto his chest. He's exhausted, though calm. Like all the fight has deserted him. 'You weren't long.'

'I can't go,' he mutters.

'I'm not surprised,' I say, preparing to transfer him back to his chair.

Is it unreasonable to expect every hospital in the country to have one toilet, equipped with ceiling hoist and changing facilities for people as disabled as Nigel? Maybe one day.

The door opens and the lovely Candia is standing there.

'There's no infection. Leave when you're ready.'

I could kiss her.

'They are coming to show you how to change the bag. Oh, here they are now,' she says pointing towards the advancing Patsy and Eddie. Hope they are more proficient in changing catheter bags than driving a mobile hoist.

Ellie and I give the two nurses as much room as possible whilst still concentrating on the technique. I'm concerned the crowding may induce a claustrophobic attack. No, his eyes are closed, his breathing is steady and his limbs are relaxed to the point of floppy. Astonishing what a cartload of Lorazepam will do.

'Now Mr Casson, would you prefer the bag strapped to your thigh, or ankle?'

'Ankle.'

'Ankle,' I repeat.

'Probably best,' she says. 'Most people prefer it out of the way.'

Patsy's trembling hands fiddle with the valves to release the drainage bag. 'Not done this for ages,' she says. 'Is this how you do it?'

You mean you don't know?

'Yes, I guess so. You lose the knack, don't you?' says Eddie.

Oh God help us. The quality manager spirit stirs within me. Demonstrations should be clear. Step by step instructions should be reinforced and understanding should be checked. This is bloody important. It's vital I do this right. 'Is there a leaflet?' I ask.

'No, sorry,' says Patsy.

Of course there isn't, that would be helpful. Are these two having a shitty day or what? They can't always be like this? Maybe it's the end of their shift and they're knackered.

'You might find something on the internet,' says Eddie.

'Right. Helpful,' I say, swallowing my irritation.

Ellie takes a photograph with her phone. That will do for now.

I am provided with a spare bag for overnight and we leave the hospital five hours after arriving.

'I need a piss!' yells Nigel the next morning.

'Oh no, what's going on?' I stare at the empty bag. This isn't right. Flapping like a demented duck, I summon the District Nurse, who happens to be a mere two streets away.

'It's on upside down,' she says, applying a new bag and alleviating Nigel's suffering.

My mistake? Or had Patsy and Eddie messed up?

23
WHEN THE LAUGHTER STOPS

July 2016

This pit is deep. He's falling. His body judders with violent, frantic spasms. He spirals downwards, pummelling against the slippery sides, plunging into the blackness. His jaw is clenched. His eyes slammed shut. His hands clasped across his chest in a formidable grip. And the shuddering goes on and on and on.

His skin is so sensitive he is unable to tolerate clothes. Ellie drapes a silk sheet over his body. He grimaces in pain as the gentle stroke of the fabric burns like acid. We open a window and direct the fan towards his face in the hope the fresh air will release the breath trapped in his throat. Olivia, the doctor from the hospice, is here, her third visit of this terrible week. I direct her to the hallway, where we speak in whispers, as the flutter of a fairy's wing might hurt his ears.

'There's nothing left to give him,' she says, reluctant to add yet more to the cocktail of thirty-seven tablets a day. 'Is he still taking Lorazepam when he's like this?'

'He had nine before I could tempt him out of bed.'

Les, who seconds ago, called in for a quick cuppa, finds himself witnessing scenes from a horror movie. 'Is there anything I can do?' he says, anxiety clouding his face.

'No, nothing,' I say. Nothing the doctor, or any of us can do. But wait. Wait for Nigel to hit the bottom of this latest pit.

A wretched whine emerges from the dining room.

'Mum,' calls Ellie.

'I need to help. Thanks for coming, Olivia.'

'Give him some extra morphine tonight,' she says.

'I'll leave now, Julie,' says Les. 'Call me if you need anything.'

'I will,' I say, knowing I won't. Les and Olivia let themselves out and I hasten to Ellie and Nigel.

Nigel is reclined in his chair, beside the open window. His entire body jerks from the onslaught of internal blows and he shivers, despite the heat. Sweat glistens on his upper lip and brow, his face flushed bright pink. Ellie, beside him, grips a damp cloth for cooling his forehead. Shimmering tears pool in her eyes.

'I don't know how to help him,' she says. 'His skin is too raw to be handled.'

I open the window wide and switch the fan to its highest setting. Its whirr will prevent Nigel from hearing the words 'We're here darling.' Undeterred, I say them anyway. He blinks in response. I motion for Ellie to join me at the table. 'We can't help him, Ellie. He'll let us know what to do when this is over.'

She nibbles at her bottom lip and watches as her dad's suffering persists. 'This one's different Mum. I don't see him coming out of this.' She closes her eyes and permits the tears to spill over. Here, in this magnificent room, a room teeming with happy memories of lavish parties, enchanting, glittering Christmases and fun-filled family gatherings, I search for understanding. How has it come to this? My precious family is broken. Smashed to pieces. As I gaze at my disease-ravaged husband and my distraught, treasured daughter I wish, with every beat of my heart, I could free them from their pain.

Perhaps Ellie's right. This one is different. The falls never last this long. He usually hits the bottom within twenty-four hours. Afterwards, there's a wait, a period of rest, before determination drives him to initiate the climb out. When at last he emerges, he is physically changed. There's a new sallowness to his complexion and the futility of his limbs has increased. The clarity of his speech has deteriorated further, his overall weakness and vulnerability enhanced. He is on a new plateau.

But he is still him. The man he has always been. The man who laughs in the face of each new disability whilst the rest of us grieve. The one who entertains his Facebook friends with his irrepressible humour and insists on recounting atrocious, corny jokes despite choking from the effort. Whose eyes twinkle with delight when surrounded by family and blaze with love when he looks at me. The man who denies MND the chance to rob him of the strength to relish every new day, to find happiness in trivia, to be grateful for his past and optimistic about his future.

I long to wrap him in my arms, to comfort him, to still the terrible trembling. What's happening to you Nigel? What horrors await you at the bottom of this pit? Will you find the courage to fight and, once again, drag yourself out? Or, is this the time, nine harrowing years on, when you accept defeat? Is this the day I fear more than any other? When MND finally conquers your unconquerable spirit? The day MND steals your laughter? Please Nig, hang on in there darling. I can't lose you yet.

Unable to endure our helplessness any longer, Ellie and I busy ourselves with whatever we can. We strip and remake Nigel's bed with clean, fresh linen. Ellie wipes the bed frame, the overbed table, the NIPPY. We freshen up his wetroom and clean the bedroom floor. The activity gives us purpose. We hope we are making a difference. Relieving the misery in some small way.

Nigel's devastated body eventually stops shuddering. Ellie stays until we succeed in tempting him to swallow a few mouthfuls of chicken soup, the one thing he can bear to consume on this torturous day, other than the morphine, which he gulps like a parched man at an oasis. We hoist him into bed, mindful not to irritate his skin with our touch, plump up his pillows and cover him with a cool cotton sheet.

Nigel spends vast amounts of time in his bedroom now. The 'West Wing', he calls it. Added around a year ago to help us stay one step ahead of his ever-increasing disability. 'It's an ensuite bedroom,' said Craig, when the building was completed, because the area is accessed via Nigel's wetroom. Yes it's odd. It's also practical. The ceiling hoist above his bed means he slides from the bed to the toilet or shower in one smooth, pain free operation. He's comfortable in here, it's become his favourite place. He watches TV as he lies in bed or looks out, through the wall of glass doors, onto the garden. I say garden, more of a yard littered with dozens of plants in pots. Still, no amount of well-placed items of elegant furniture, or gallery of photographs and paintings lining the walls, transform it from being anything other than what it is: a private ward.

The morphine has done its job. Nigel is sound asleep. His chest rises and falls as the NIPPY, whooshing like Darth Vader, directs air into his lungs through the tube attached to the nose pillow tucked in his nostrils, and secured by a strap around his head. It must be uncomfortable. I'm reminded of the recent selfie he posted on Facebook strapped up like this. 'This gets right up my bloody nose,' he'd written. I check the catheter drainage bag hanging from the bed frame. Yes, that should last until morning. The catheter, now a permanent solution, has provided at least some relief from the constant need to be close to a toilet. I place the battery for the mobile hoist in its charging station, make sure the bed is plugged in and the remote within his reach, check the degree of charge in his iPad and lay out his morning medication. Lastly, I draw the sheet under his chin and place a tender kiss on his cheek.

I won't leave him alone tonight, I need to be with him. Resting in the riser recliner in the corner of the bedroom, acquired for the comfort of the carer on the overnight shift, I prepare for a sleepless night. Phone, Kindle, pinot. Bodger hops onto the chair and wriggles into the gap at my side. 'We'll look after him, Bodge,' I whisper, stroking his soft, velvety coat. 'You and me. We're his carers tonight.' Bodger harrumphs in the way dogs do and snuggles deeper into the gap, his eyes closed. 'OK, just me then.'

I pour a glass of wine and study my sleeping husband. Where have your dreams taken you, Nig? Are you in your wheelchair when you dream nowadays? Or has MND robbed you of your dreams as well? Are you free of it when you sleep? Do you still run and climb and ride your bike and erect complex scaffold structures? Maybe the morphine has mixed things up a bit and you're zipping along the scaffold boards in your chair, performing elaborate wheelies. You'd love that.

Perhaps you're playing golf? Eating up the sun-baked courses on the Costa del Sol, displaying skills akin to Seve's, or thrashing around with your mates here in Scarborough. Do you sense the swish of the driver as you strike the ball, connecting with the sweet spot of the clubface, watching it soar like a bullet to land an easy three hundred yards away slap bang in the centre of the fairway? Are you judging your approach with a chip shot, mastering the bounce and roll of the ball as it hits the green? Or nailing the perfect rhythm of the delicate putting stroke and sinking the ball like a pro?

You could be in the Indigo. Leaning on the bar, pint in hand, discussing the day's business with Glyn. Those jobs stripped, those erected. What's coming up next? Who's paid, who hasn't? Which of the lads failed to show up, which gang could carry more work? You share a joke with the landlord and order another round. 'One for yourself, mate,' you say as Graham pulls your pint of real ale. He's delighted. 'Thank you, sir! You're a Gent.'

Or are you with me? Where are we? What are we doing?

Is it our wedding day? You, with your horseshoe moustache and cropped black hair, the Elvis quiff already a thing of the past. Resplendent in your smart battleship grey, straight off the peg, Burton suit. Silver tie fashioned in full Windsor knot the size of your chin and Cuban heel platform boots. Me, dressed like a princess in the gown Mum created, white satin with hanging sleeves. Borrowed pearl choker, pearl earrings and pearl-tipped tiara. Are you waiting as I walk down the aisle towards you? We shivered in that vast, freezing, church for over an hour. I remember thinking our guests would hate us.

I bet you've swept me onto the dance floor to twirl to Van Morrison's *Brown Eyed Girl*. You'd never allow me to remain seated when that song came on. I close my eyes and attempt to summon the memory of the last time Nigel held me in his arms as we danced. 'What was the occasion, Nig? Where was it? It seems a long time ago.' I recall the first time, however: that engagement do at Whitcliffe Mount. I asked you to dance with me to avoid the unwelcome advances of some lad. What was his name? It doesn't matter, he gave me the excuse to talk to you. We had our first kiss that night. You said you'd ring me on Friday to arrange a night out. You never did, you bugger. So, I chased you. Not letting you escape so easily.

Are we on holiday in Malta, melting in the sun or keeping cool in the pool? God it was hot. I spent the entire time covered in calamine lotion, in the hope of soothing the sunspots. You and Craig couldn't stop laughing at the state of me. Or maybe Tenerife. That bloody awful hotel? I wept all day. We vowed, then, to up the quality of accommodation in future. How did we end up in that shitty apartment in Florida? Disney made up for it though, didn't it, Nig? Can you picture the delight on Ellie and Becky's faces as they marvelled at the awe-inspiring, endless procession of Disney's characters? Craig loved it too: the piano player, in particular, held him captivated by his rendition of 'The Entertainer'. How many hundreds of times has Craig since belted out that tune?

I reach for the bottle of pinot at the side of the chair and refill my glass. Nigel hasn't stirred in over an hour. Where are you now, Nig? What's happening inside your head? Are the things you've done, places you've seen, whizzing around in a maelstrom of disjointed memories? Are you wandering along the Champs d'Elysees in Paris, or cleaning windows with Craig? You could be cleaning windows along the Champs d'Elysees. Who knows? You may be driving us all to Scarborough in that rickety old Transit van. What hope we had. What ambition. You might be swinging from the scaffolding on the Thelwall Viaduct above the Manchester Ship Canal. Or singing 'Old Mother Lee' in the bath. The grandchildren might be opening their presents on Christmas morning. It wouldn't surprise me if you're hurtling headfirst towards the tarmac as Ellie and her bike collide catastrophically into yours. You could be in Vegas, winning a few dollars. Well, losing, considering your record. Win or lose, who cares?

Wherever you are, I miss you. Awfully. I miss us. I miss the life we had and mourn our ransacked future. We never expected this, did we, Nig? We never dreamt we'd end up where we are right now.

I drain and refill my glass, disturbing Bodger as I reach for my phone. He leaps from the chair and curls up at my feet. 'Sorry, Bodge.'

Clicking on the Facebook icon, a notification from Tracey pops up. Oh, another of those motivational quotes. She loves this kind of stuff. Dalai Lama values, inspirational songs, yoga. No matter what befalls her she'll find a reason to be optimistic and trust that whatever happens, happens for a reason. Nevertheless, she does tend to pop along to a medium every so often, to make sure she's on the right track.

> 'Learn from yesterday,
> Live for today,
> Hope for tomorrow.'
> *Albert Einstein*

Ah Tracey, noble sentiment indeed. I'm reluctant to add my own 'like' to the 1.4k others and mumble instead, 'Yeah, yeah, whatever, Trace.' We've had a fair crack at all that. This journey of Nigel's has taught us heaps about life, living and hope. Especially you Nig. What did you say when you passed the five-year mark? 'Every day is a bonus.' And since then, you have embraced each unexpected day with courage, laughter and love. We treasure our days, don't we? We do. You transcend the misery far better than I. You are the bravest man I know. The only inspiration I will ever need.

Yet I question, gazing at Nigel lying in his bed, having shared his excruciating day, if living for today is an option anymore, now all his todays are as shit as this one? I make the mistake of clicking on the comments tab and am bombarded with, 'You never know what's round the corner.' 'Life is a gift, treasure it.' 'Live every day as if it's your last.' Ha, that's a classic. We've all vowed to do that at some point. When the curtain closes on the coffin of a loved one, that's when you determine to get the best out of life. Filing out of the crematorium, the plot to conquer death takes shape. Death won't sneak up on me before I'm damn well ready, goes the rant. I will not die harbouring regret. I will make sure I say and do everything I need to. Not another minute will I waste. I will welcome each day with joy. I will live every day as if it's my last.

I've dismissed those good intentions by the time I raise a glass to toast the dead. I mean, how would it work in practice? Would I linger more as I walk Bodger? Would I hold my face to the rain as I do to the sun? Chat with fellow dog-walkers? Remark on the splendid day, the swell of the sea, the tranquil sky? Would I actually walk the dog? Yes, of course. Couldn't die with that kind of guilt. On my last day, who would I choose to see? Who would I exclude? Perhaps I might take a moment to lounge on one of the many benches on the Esplanade, read its memorial plaque and ponder on the lives of those already loved and lost. I could share their beloved view of Scarborough for a while.

'Would you like a bench, Nig? On the golf course, perhaps?' I reach for the bottle of pinot and refill my glass. Sliding down well, this. Is that such a stupid idea? I explore the notion as I sip my drink. It should be on the eighth tee, with the plaque reading: 'Advice from the late David Nigel Casson: "Don't drive into that clump of trees on the right."' You'd howl at that. On reading those words their drive would slice straight into Casson's Copse. So thoughtful of the Club to name that clump of trees after you. Not surprising, given your drives landed there every single time.

'Cass, you bastard!' they'll say, and snigger as their memories are revived.

As the image of a group of golfers heading towards Casson's Copse, chuckling at their memories, swamps my mind, I clamp my fist over my mouth to strangle the rising sob in my throat. Oh God, listen to me. You're not dead yet, and I've bought you a bloody bench.

Nigel stirs. I tip forward ready to jump up if he wakes, fist still fastened to my face. He shifts his head in search of a soft spot on the pillow, and settles, grimacing behind eyes screwed shut. Did you read my mind? I'm sorry darling. Forget the bench. There'll be no more talk of a bench. I hold my breath. Wait. Listen to the rhythm of the NIPPY forcing air into his lungs. After a moment, his features relax and the fine creases around his eyes soften as slumber steals him away. It's OK. I sink back in the chair, relieved. Must be my imagination. Bodger wriggles at my feet, exhales a drowsy harrumph and rolls onto his other side. The pair of them should sleep like the dead until tomorrow.

'And what of tomorrow?' I ask, as I down the last of the wine. What will that give us? As sure as hell it won't be hope. Not for me anyway. How do you feel, Nig? Is there any hope for tomorrow left in you? Could you tolerate another tomorrow as horrendous as today?

I am weary of this dreadful day and yearn for it to be over. Exhausted, my entire body screams for rest. I rub my aching shoulders and rotate my head to relieve the tension in my neck. The action resembles a pestle grinding cardamon pods in a mortar, so I stop. Reclining the chair to its limit, I give up the fight and I allow my stinging eyes to close. Ten minutes should do it. Maybe half an hour. An hour, max.

A low, rumbling growl drags me awake. Something's wrong. The room is cloaked in darkness. Nigel's outline in his bed and the whoosh of the NIPPY tells me he is still sleeping. Bodger is on his feet. I peer through the glass to the garden. An intruder? I can't discern anything outside. It's never like this in July. Pulling my dressing gown tight around me, I jerk up and reach for my phone. It will soon be dawn. It should be light. The seagulls should be screeching by now. 'What is it Bodge?' I whisper. 'What's happening?' He stares at Nigel's bed, growling deep inside his throat. A long, threatening grumble which ends, without warning, in a startled yap. He drops to the floor, tucks his head in his paws. What the –?

'Ah.' The old enemy. That ethereal spectre of Death hovers at the end of Nigel's bed. 'You again.'

I lift Bodger from the floor and pitch him in the chair. He doesn't resist.

'What do you want?' I ask of the thing. I said all there was to say last time it showed up. I'm bored of it now. 'We're not frightened of you,' I continue. 'There's nothing you can do to hurt us.'

The phantom appears different somehow. Not as vile. Not dripping with disgusting decay. Tonight, it doesn't lay its putrid hand upon him. Instead, one arm extends above Nigel's body, palm upwards. The other arm reaches out to me, open and welcoming. I don't understand. Where is the usual menace? Where's the evil smirk?

There is no contempt in what could be called its face. Wow. I don't believe it. This apparition, this ghoul I never gave a name, the thing which has assaulted my consciousness again and again, is looking at me with unmistakable compassion.

The squawk of caterwauling seagulls in search of breakfast wakes me. When I prize open my eyes they're so full of grit I'm sure I slept on the beach. The garden glows like fire and is awash with sunshine. I stretch my neck and halt as cardamon pods crunch. Bodger is at my feet. The TV is on. Nigel has inclined his bed.

'Good morning, darling,' he says. 'Any chance of a cuppa?'

24

IT'S ALL ABOUT CONTROL

August 2016

The days following Nigel's rise from the pit are as serene as the former were frenzied, and a welcome, if fragile, tranquillity pervades our home. I tiptoe from room to room, taking measured, silent steps, lest a sudden clamour – a trip, a dropped cup – should provoke the demons and reignite Nigel's internal torture.

As is always the case, he is physically changed. The incident has weakened him further. Like air squeezed from a balloon, the last lingering pockets of strength desert him and leave him deflated. This man, who thought nothing of carrying two 13' scaffold boards on a single shoulder, hasn't the strength to lift his toothbrush.

Yet the astounding transformation is the disappearance of the all-consuming anxiety. His little helpers, those calming Lorazepam tablets he devours like smarties, remain untouched. Until now, these tiny blue orbs of pure magic are the reason he tolerates each passing hour, the enabler for a doctor's or family member's visit, the armour protecting him from the anticipation of painful spasms, the reinforcements for leaving the house and the remedy for insomnia. The fretful snatches of drug-induced oblivion are now replaced by periods of deep, restful sleep. When not sleeping, he is composed, in control of his previously tormented psyche and at peace with his lot.

'What's happening Nig?' I ask, retrieving the six discarded Lorazepam tablets from the side table and holding them in my palm. 'Don't need these anymore?'

Reclined in his chair, he glances at the tablets and a slow grin brightens his pallid face. 'You've clocked it.'

'Hard not to. The change in you.'

He raises his eyebrows and hunches his shoulders like he's guarding a secret.

'You won the lottery or something?'

'Ha,' he laughs. 'Better than that.'

'OK. What?'

He squints at me, as though contemplating whether he can trust me. Should he share the miracle which occurred when my back was turned? With studied deliberation, he adjusts the riser recliner until he's upright. The action signifies the importance of what he's about to say and I'm compelled to perch on the edge of the settee.

Shining more blue than green today, the bleak, troubled expression in those striking eyes, which has haunted him for months, is gone, and something new is reflected there. What am I seeing? Perplexed, I search his face. Is it resolve? No, it's more than that.

'I've found the cure,' he says.

In a flash, I recognise the expression. He's triumphant.

What cure? There is no cure. There is but one way to be free of MND. He knows that. Why is he grinning like he expects to tear open a gift and find all he ever craved in the box? As I gaze at the face I love, a splinter of fear pierces my consciousness and in that second, I grasp, with absolute certainty, what he intends to do. At once, it all makes sense. His calm demeanour, the disregarded Lorazepam, the relaxing sleep. Knowing the answer already, I ask anyway.

'What do you mean?'

I wait. He takes a deep breath and, in a voice, as powerful and unwavering as is possible when defiled by disease, says, 'I'm going to Dignitas.'

Is it possible to be not at all surprised and yet stunned at the same time? Part of me expected this. Hearing those words, spoken with such resolve, punches a hole in my core and I fall back against the cushions with a gasp. I am transported to the night following Nigel's diagnosis, when we spent the hours before dawn scouring the internet, devouring every morsel we could find on MND, as we sought an explanation, a means to understand why this was happening. Link after link of this complex labyrinth we pursued in our quest to secure that elusive roadmap leading to a cure. Something, anything to inspire us, to raise our spirits, to give us hope. That night, we discovered Craig Ewart, a man suffering from motor neurone disease, who travelled with his wife to Dignitas in Switzerland to end his life. Together, we watched him draw his final breath.

'Poor man,' I said.

'Not a bad way to go,' said Nigel.

And then, soon afterwards, when speaking to the kids, he joked, 'There's always Dignitas.'

There's been no mention of Dignitas since. I wonder if Nigel's planned this all along? A way to end it. At a time of his choosing.

'Are you sure?' I ask.

A stupid question, I know. Of course he's sure. This is not a decision made lightly, like choosing meat or fish from the menu. Or one of those outcomes determined by the toss of a coin. This is serious. Deadly serious.

The effort of sitting upright exhausts him and he reclines his chair and rests his head on the smooth fabric, as a murmur of assent resonates in his throat. The triumphant glimmer in his eyes now fades to a shadowy fusion of sorrowful acceptance, and the spectre of Death, our unwelcome companion for ten years, weighs heavily upon his collapsed body.

Not once, in our struggle on this treacherous journey, when at times our defences have been crushed by the merciless cruelty we encounter and at others, where laughter has been our champion, have we discussed what happens when we reach the end of this road.

Nigel challenges the devastating effects of this dreadful disease with awe-inspiring guts and gritty humour. 'The laughing Grandad,' young Tom calls him. So true. His legendary hilarity has echoed throughout our home. He has stuck two fingers up at this invincible enemy. Until, that is, the laughter stopped. When, two months ago, the plateau upon which he felt secure crumbled beneath him, plunging him to the depths of that final pit. What terrors assaulted him there? What anguish did he endure? What changed for him to long for the mercy of death?

I kneel beside Nigel's chair. Clasping one shrunken hand in both of mine I press my lips to the satiny, translucent skin, so far removed from those oil-blackened, bone-crushing paws of his youth. 'Have you had all you can take, Nig?' I whisper. 'Can't you bear anymore?'

The intense love swirling in those captivating eyes chokes me. I try to suppress the sob as I press my lips to his hand but it erupts anyway.

'It's not what I can bear,' he stutters.

'What is it?'

'I've no control any more,' he says.

'Control?'

Nigel heaves a sigh, searching for the words to express his thoughts. 'Yes. It's beating me.'

'Never.'

'Yes Julie, it is.'

With the fragment of strength he has left, he raises a trembling arm and touches my cheek before his hand flops to my shoulder. He draws a long, determined breath and with quiet, steady tones, says, 'But I won't let it. I know it will annihilate me if I don't stop it. I won't give it the pleasure. I need to get in first.'

The set of his chin tells me he means it. My husband, the warrior, has never deserted. He remains inside that body. Though this adversary, this MND, has defeated him in many battles, Nigel will be the ultimate victor in this ruinous war. He is taking control. As he always has. This is how he's managed each debilitating physical disability from the outset. The wheelchair purchased before he couldn't walk. No more than two guests at a time. Wetroom ready prior to him needing it. Carers interviewed and on the team. Bedroom extension built. Equipment in place and ready to operate. These acts of preparation, some minor, some immense, combine to ensure his sense of control. This is what empowers him to influence his life, his daily routine, his happiness.

'I understand,' I whisper, the words lost against the hammering of my heart.

'Do you?' he says, with some urgency. 'Do you really understand?'

I squeeze his hand. 'Yes, I do. Truly, I do.'

His eyes close, his head lolls back and he sinks into the chair. His body shudders as the tension leaves.

'I must make this choice, Julie,' he says. 'While I still can.'

'I know, my darling.'

'The disease is changing me. I won't let it make me disappear.'

I contemplate the absent joyfulness. The increased and lengthy panic attacks. The non-existent socialising. The growing dependence on pills and the gulping of gallons of morphine. The supremacy over his body is already accomplished. That battle is over. The campaign to deprive him of his resolve and sense of self has begun. No. He's right. It must not be allowed to happen.

'You could never disappear.'

'I could. I am. I know it. This is my one chance to stop it.'

'I understand, Nig.'

Encouraged, he relaxes into his chair. I shuffle closer to him and rest my head on his thigh. He strokes my hair.

'Do you remember what the Professor said?' he says. 'It never changes pace?'

'Yes.'

'I could be buried alive for years. Unable to drag a scream from my throat.'

The image of Nigel trapped inside a shattered body, with a mind astute and attuned to his surroundings, forced to endure unimaginable torture, unable to express his wishes, share his thoughts or cry for help, overwhelms me, and silent tears slide down my face. Should he be condemned to a living hell, where he longs for each new day to be his last? What anguish would I witness reflected in his eyes? Could I stand by as his spirit is sucked out of him? Must he suffer month after month, year after year, desperate for the moment his breathing stops, until finally, he is granted the release only death provides?

'Hey,' he says, wiping my tears, 'You've drenched my leg.'

'Sorry,' I sniff.

The flicker of his smile as he cups my chin pierces my soul. It is filled with both contentment and melancholy.

'I want to die while I'm happy,' he says. 'While I can still smile.'

I make no attempt to stem the tears as I draw him into my arms.

'Oh Nig, I love you so much.'

Pressing his face to my chest, locked within my embrace, for only the second time since his diagnosis, he allows himself to weep.

25
APPLY TO DIE

The niggling question, 'How to transport Nigel to Switzerland?' is placed in the 'deal with it later box' with the lid slammed shut and the key chucked to the back of the bit drawer inside my head. Nevertheless, the complexity of the task escapes its internment to prod at me like a persistent bully with a stick. I mean, according to Google, it's 865 miles from Scarborough to Zurich. When did Nigel last venture as far as the end of the street? He hasn't left the house in months, and when he does, it demands military operational planning. 'No problem there, Julie,' I say, once again ramming the nagging issue back in the box. My platoon is teeming with military folk. When the time comes, we'll sort it. The priority right now, is Dignitas.

Dignitas is one of those places people have heard of yet know nothing about. Gaps in knowledge are filled with made up nonsense and repeatedly exuded until it's regarded as true. So, to smash one such myth: Dignitas is not a clinic. According to its excellent website, it is a not-for-profit member's society which supports self-determination, autonomy and dignity. It's mission statement: 'To live with dignity – to die with dignity' is as concerned with life's choices as it is with choice at life's end. You can't rock up uninvited and ask to be put out of one's misery, it's nothing like that simple. Furthermore, whilst Dignitas supports assisted and accompanied suicide, it is actively engaged in suicide attempt prevention.

This particular website, along with a plethora of articles written on Dignitas, and countless videos on YouTube of people who made the journey, consume our afternoons, once the carers leave, and we are free to pursue our research in secret. For now, secrecy is paramount.

First, a fee of 200 Swiss francs is required for Nigel to become a member. You don't need to be terminally ill, you may not be contemplating suicide, you may join if you simply share the organisation's values. If, like Nigel, you happen to be applying to access the service of accompanied suicide, there are several prerequisites, including the need for unassailable judgement and sufficient physical mobility to administer the drug yourself.

'I knew this would come in handy,' says Nigel, lifting his T-shirt to expose the gastric tube. 'I'll take the drug through this.'

'They've to accept you yet, Nig. You've to be of sound mind as well, don't forget.'

'Ha ha. Funny. What else?'

'Let's see. Well, being pissed off isn't good enough. You must suffer from one or more of the following. Number one, a terminal illness.'

'Got.'

'Unendurable, incapacitating disability.'

'Got.'

'Unbearable, uncontrollable pain.'

'Sometimes got. I qualify on at least two and a half counts, I reckon,' says Nigel. 'Piece of piss.'

'It's not as easy as that,' I say, reading on.

'What?'

'You've to write a letter giving the reason you're requesting accompanied suicide, your physical condition and how it affects you.'

'OK. Not difficult.'

'No, it's not. They also need a bucketload of medical reports, full case history from diagnosis, the treatment you've received, medication, prognosis and so on. Old reports and bang up to date ones.'

'All in the file,' he says. 'Where is it?'

'I'll find it.'

I race to the cupboard in the hall where I keep the tome of documents I wish we didn't possess. The MNDA file is in there, a membership gift from when Nigel joined this particular club back in 2007. There beside it, is a red foolscap, push button box file, containing GP referrals and hospital appointments Nigel has attended, along with subsequent specialist reports involved in the diagnosis, and Olivia's records of on-going treatment and deteriorating condition, dating from last month to way back, when Brenda wrote her report on Nigel's pesky plosives.

'Will it cover it?' says Nigel.

'I don't know. I'll check. You need to talk to Doctor Brown and Olivia, regardless.'

'I intend to.'

'Great.'

'Is that it?' he says, indicating the Dignitas website on my laptop.

'No.'

'What's left?'

'They require a biography describing your childhood, school life, family circumstances and the primary events in your life.'

'Bloody hell.'

'Indeed. And also, details of who supports your request for accompanied suicide.'

'Right.'

'And, who will be travelling with you to Switzerland.'

'OK,' he says, extending his hand for me to grasp. 'I take it you are?'

'Naturally.'

He releases my hand and points to the photograph of Craig, Ellie and Becky smiling back at us, taken with my phone at Craig's 40th. 'I'd better speak to the kids. Ask if they fancy a trip to Zurich.'

...

Ellie hears the news the next day whilst carrying out her morning caring routine. Out of bed, showered and breakfasted, he tells her as she massages his feet, an indulgence he relishes daily.

'I'm not surprised,' she says. 'If anything, I suppose I was expecting it, after your last episode. You mentioned Dignitas, right after your diagnosis, didn't you? Never since.'

'Yes. Until now. It's time.'

'I understand, Daddylumps,' she says, kissing his big toe.

'Will you come with us?'

'Yes, I'll come,' she says. 'Wouldn't let you go alone. You'll need me. Mum couldn't manage you on her own.'

Becky, due home from the the Netherlands in a few weeks, to take up her post at the Ministry of Defence, hears from me over the phone, as usual.

'Ah, poor Dad,' she says, after taking a moment to process my explanation that Dad regards this as his cure. 'He must be ready to make that choice. I'm so glad he can.'

'Will you come with us?'

'Are you kidding? Of course. When do I book leave?'

'Not yet, no date agreed yet.'

'OK. Let me know soon as, and I'll sort it.'

She'll hide in her bed and cry now, I suspect, as I end the call.

Nigel announces his proposed cure to Craig when he pops in to entertain us with achingly funny accounts of his morning's tribulations. The old woman in the shop who takes half an hour to unbuckle her handbag, find the compartment containing her purse, unzip, no, wrong compartment, zip, unzip the next. Purse located, unzip. 'Oh, there's a voucher in here somewhere. Yes, here it is.' Pops it on the counter. 'How much is it again?' Takes out a fiver, fiddles for the change, clocks she's short of money. 'I'll pay with my card. Now, where is it?'

'What time do you close?' says Craig, fidgeting in the queue.

Or the fella who asks him if he does flat windows.

'Yes, and curved ones.'

The customer who calls him a miserable bastard because he insists on taking the Christmas tree down on Boxing Day, or the lady who, like him, knows the words to 'Chattanooga Choo Choo' and sings along as he plays his keyboard, which he keeps in his van, for when it rains.

It doesn't matter if we've heard it all before, his tales brighten Nigel's day.

'Fuck me,' he says. 'That's some cure.'

I hand him a cup of tea, which he sips in silence, contemplating the enormity of the news. During these ten years, we've grown so accustomed to Nigel's illness it is difficult to contemplate a different existence. It's easy to be lulled into believing these days will never end.

'When?' Craig says, eventually.

'We don't know yet. Your dad has to write to Dignitas and send a load of bumf. Then, if they agree, they'll issue the green light. Could take a couple of months. A date won't be set until then.'

'A couple of months?'

'Yes, maybe three.'

'It's like when you told us the diagnosis.'

'Sorry,' says Nigel. 'Will you come with us?'

Craig scrubs his face with his hands, as if attempting to rearrange his features. He screws his eyes shut, sniffs and clamps his lips between his teeth. Then, drawing a long, controlled breath, says, 'Well, you won't have MND anymore, Dad.'

'Exactly,' says Nigel.

'Another cuppa?' I suggest, hoping this will give Craig time to answer his dad's question.

'Yes, why not,' says Craig. 'A cup of tea fixes everything doesn't it?'

'No. That's wine,' I say, filling the kettle.

I must make at least thirty cups of tea a day. I buy teabags by the thousand from Bookers, along with dozens of paper cups, lids and straws Nigel needs to drink the stuff.

Following the restorative brew, two shortbread, three chocolate biscuits and a tale of some twat moaning about Craig's van being parked on the pavement outside Pizza Hut, Craig says, 'What about the police?'

'What about 'em?' says Nigel.

'Don't they stop people from going to Dignitas?'

'Er, maybe, if they know about it. I believe the police prevented two sisters from raising funds to take their mum to Dignitas. Last year, I think.' I say. 'They got her there in the end though.'

'What was wrong with her?'

'MND.'

'Yeah, what else?' he says. And, as if searching for reasons to scupper the plan, 'What happens when we come home? Will there be an investigation?'

'I honestly don't know,' I reply. 'Anyway, I suspect they'd focus on me, not you three.'

'I can't do with the coppers interviewing me.'

'That's why we're only telling certain people,' Nigel explains. 'Just close family, Doctor Brown and Olivia from the hospice. Maybe a couple of trusted friends.'

'I wouldn't trust any bugger.'

Nigel says, 'You don't need to come, you know Craig. Don't feel pressured.'

I force myself to keep my mouth shut. Yes, he does. He'd regret it for the rest of his life, if he didn't.

'It's OK if you don't want to.'

No, it bloody isn't OK. I chew the inside of my bottom lip and resist the urge to shove a gag in Nigel's mouth. 'Why don't you give it some thought?' I suggest. 'There's still time.'

'No, I don't need to think,' he says. ''Course I'm coming. Try stopping me.'

Never doubted it for a moment.

•••

Later that night, as Ellie and I prepare Nigel for bed, he says, 'You know, Craig might have a point.'

'What do you mean?' I ask.

'A police investigation when you come back to Scarborough. I'd hate that to happen.'

'Why would it?' says Ellie, freeing one arm from his lounge-wear top.

'Assisted suicide's illegal in the UK,' he says.

'I know, that's why you're off to Switzerland.'

'Yes, but they could still question you all.'

Ellie attaches the sling to the ceiling hoist while I remove the duvet and plump up the pillow. 'Don't care if they do,' she says.

'At risk of appearing pedantic,' I say. 'You're not planning *assisted* suicide. It's *accompanied* suicide. Assisted is when a doctor or somebody else gives you the lethal drug. Accompanied is when you do it yourself and people are with you. Massively different.'

Ellie grabs her phone. 'Mmm, not as clear cut as you might think, when you Google it. Type in *accompanied suicide* and *assisted* pops up.'

'Well, whatever, Nig love, don't worry your head. We'll be prepared in case there's an investigation. We'll know what to say. It'll be fine.'

'Maybe I should make a video,' he says.

Ellie and I exchange puzzled glances.

'What kind of video?'

'To prove I'm acting of my own free will. Confirm I've done all the preparation myself and nobody has coerced me.'

'Bloody hell, Nig.'

'In case we'd talked you into killing yourself because you're a bloody nuisance?' says Ellie.

'Yeah.'

'Shit, we'd better fix this story, Mum.'

Nigel sniggers and gestures for Ellie to pass his cup.

'Please stop worrying, Nig. Make a video if you like. Although, when you talk to the doctor and Olivia they will add the information to your medical records.'

'That's true,' he says, relaxing. 'I'll mention it next week.'

He leans back against the pillow. 'Come on, shove this NIPPY on me.'

'Ey, wait a minute you,' says Ellie, holding the nose pillow away from his face. 'Did you ask Craig and Becky if they'd pay for you to go to Dignitas, like you asked me?'

'You what?' I say.

Nigel looks sheepish. 'No.'

'What?'

He chuckles.

'Only me was it?'

'What's so funny, Nig?'

'When he told me about going to Dignitas, he said if he couldn't afford it, would I pay for him?'

'You cheeky bugger.'

Nigel's giggling prevents Ellie from fitting the NIPPY around his head. 'Love test wasn't it?' she says. 'Now stop laughing and let me ram this on your bloody head.'

When at last he's settled into bed, Ellie kisses one cheek, I kiss the other.

''Night, darling. Don't worry.'

''Night, Dad. And yes, I would pay.'

'I knew it. 'Night girls. Love you.'

'Love you too,' we echo, as we leave his bedroom and head for the kitchen.

'Pinot?'

•••

226

If the pitiful Dianne Pretty had won the right for her husband or doctor to help her die; if the campaign for 'Dignity in Dying' had already succeeded in convincing Parliament, the Lords and the Church that the majority of the population of this country believe terminally ill adults should be granted control and choice over how they die, then assisted suicide would be legal and Nigel would not need to contemplate travelling to Zurich to end his life. As it is, any person helping another commit suicide faces up to fourteen years in prison. This may explain why dying Britons who travel to Dignitas – an astonishing one every eight days – fail to announce their intentions in advance.

Dying a horrible, lingering, painful death isn't enough for this country. Add on the gruelling journey, to be taken before the poor sods are unable to travel, the not insignificant expense, anywhere between £6,500 to £15,000, and mix it up with the profound anxiety of what may happen to accompanying family members. This all forces plans to be shrouded in secrecy and innocent people to behave like criminals and to die sooner than needed.

'The law makes you sick, doesn't it?' I say, handing a generous glass of pinot to Ellie.

'Cheers,' she says. 'Yes, it's insane. It has to change one day.'

'Not in time for your dad, though.'

'No.' She takes a sip. 'Any idea how we get to Switzerland?'

'God knows. I daren't contemplate it yet. Let's wait until he's been given the green light. Once we have it, we'll fret about that.'

We finish the bottle before Ellie heads home and Jeanette arrives for the nightshift.

•••

The latest file I wish we didn't possess is a bright red A4 ring binder, bursting with empty plastic pockets waiting to be filled. Nigel sets up a Dignitas folder on his email account and the process is underway.

The letter holding the power to grant Nigel his wish to be in control of his death, is composed.

'Dear Sir or Madam

Membership No: 255.54.391

'I am writing to make a request for an accompanied suicide with the help of Dignitas. I was diagnosed with Motor Neurone Disease in 2007 and have since suffered a slow and continuous deterioration of my physical mobility and speech.

'The disease has now progressed to a point where I need constant care and I am unable to do most things without help. I am unable to walk, stand, move position, or attend to any of my personal needs. I need to be hoisted into my wheelchair and bed and onto the toilet.

'Whilst my mobility is severely impaired, I still have movement in my hands and arms. I still swallow and manage a diet of soft food, although I have a PEG tube, which, at this stage, is for administering medication. I have a catheter. I rely on a non-invasive ventilator to assist with breathing overnight and increasingly during the day.

'I take a significant amount of medication, a lot of it prescribed to combat the pain and discomfort associated with my physical condition and the spasms in my limbs, and also to alleviate the constant anxiety and distress, as I lose more and more control of my body.

'I have had a wonderful life that I am happy to have shared with my supportive and loving wife and children. Before my diagnosis,

I was an active and fit individual. I was a director of two successful construction businesses, travelled extensively and enjoyed a busy social life. I played golf, cycled and supported my local rugby club.

'I am a naturally cheerful person and have tried to maintain my sense of humour and good spirits even as this disease has progressed and changed my working and family life to the extent where I can no longer participate in any of the things I love.

'I have now reached the point where my condition is unendurable. I know motor neurone disease will continue to ravage what is left of my body. I know it will be a slow and torturous process. Ultimately, I will be unable to move and unable to speak. I will be trapped in a helpless body without the ability to communicate my frustration or desires. The physical and mental agony this will cause me, not to mention the anguish and pain for my family, is intolerable to me.

'I am proud and pleased to leave my wife and children in a financially secure situation. They have brought me endless joy and I love them with all my heart. But it is time for me to leave.

'I am not afraid of dying. I would welcome it. I would like to exercise one final act of control in my life and die whilst I am still smiling.'

I print the letter, add it to the 'Patient's Instructions' form required by Dignitas on becoming a member, and four medical reports dating from 2008 to 2016 along with the biographical sketch of his life, family and next of kin.

'I want to ask Dignitas some questions,' he says. 'I'll add it to that lot.'

'What are they?'

'Can I stay in the wheelchair to take the drug?'

'Given that stepping out of it isn't an option, I would hope so.'

'What happens to the chair once I'm dead?'

'Ah, no surprise there. Is that because it cost more than our first house? You don't want it dumped?'

'Damn right. It could be donated to a hospice or something.'

'Of course. Anymore?'

'If a syringe is inserted in the PEG tube do I push it myself or what? Tidy the words up a bit. You know what I mean.'

'No problem.'

'That'll do.'

'Er, wait a minute,' I say. 'What about bringing your body home? Shouldn't you ask for info on that?'

I fix him with a stern stare. The tilt of his head and whisper of a pitying smile says, 'Now come on, don't make a fuss, let it be.'

'It's not that easy, you know, Julie. I don't mind what happens to me afterwards.'

'You care more for your chair than your own body.'

'It's not that,' he insists. 'It's not a service Dignitas offers.'

I'm tempted to ask how he knows that? Which snippet of information has he read that I've missed? I bite my tongue and settle for, 'Well, ask, eh?'

'Fair enough,' he says. 'I'll ask.'

I collate all the documents and create a cover sheet identifying the contents in the pack. I make copies, slot them into plastic wallets and add them to the red file along with Nigel's membership form, and print-outs of each email, arranged in date order, sent and received so far. I place the originals in a padded envelope to be sent by registered post the following morning. My secretarial college lecturer would be proud of me.

And now, we wait. Albeit not patiently. Nigel insists I track the parcel's progress daily. It's still in England. It's on the plane. It's landed. It's in Switzerland. In Zurich. Delivered. When Nigel is alerted by the clattering of the letterbox, I am sent scurrying to retrieve the post. Is it them? Have they answered? Nineteen days later, on 28 August 2016, a premium quality, latte tinted envelope hits the mat.

I bear this critical sachet to Nigel's bedroom as if nursing a wounded butterfly. 'It's here.'

Nigel adjusts the controls of his bed and raises himself up. 'Open it.'

I do so, reverently, and extract a matching latte piece of superior paper, embellished with the Dignitas logo, centred at the top of the page, in green. I hold the document and lean close beside him so we can read it together.

'Fuck,' I say, on reaching the second paragraph. 'A psychiatric statement? Wasn't expecting that.'

The letter states that, as Nigel is taking Citalopram and Lorazepam, they must be sure his decisional capacity is not influenced by anxiety or medication, and a psychiatric statement is required. Our questions are not answered. They take a step-by-step approach, and these will be discussed later, it says. Next step, provide the required psychiatric report. An invoice for a special membership contribution of 3,500 Swiss francs will follow, and Nigel's case will be submitted to one of their collaborating physicians for consideration. Once Nigel receives the 'provisional green light', which means the physician provisionally agrees to write the prescription for the lethal drug, we move to the next stage.

'Right,' says Nigel. 'Better find a shrink.'

This proves more difficult than one might imagine. Doctor Brown refers us to a local psychiatrist who, on learning Nigel's intentions, flatly refuses to speak to him. A second psychiatrist does the same. Not wishing to increase Nigel's anxiety level any more than this setback already has, I restrict my outraged rant to, 'Opinionated bastards. How dare they make judgement before they've spoken to you?'

Could this signal the end of Nigel's hopes for Dignitas? Will the lack of one simple report condemn him to suffer a wretched, intolerable existence? No way. He mustn't let that happen. The search for an open-minded private psychiatric doctor with no such scruples leads us to York, and a third referral is made on Nigel's behalf. Given his degree of immobility, this enlightened individual agrees to come to Scarborough to assess Nigel at home.

'Like I've said before, I'm glad we're not skint,' he says, when I tell him her fee. The truth is, no amount of money would be considered excessive for Nigel to secure this report.

'Try to behave like you're right in the head,' I say, heading to answer the door to Dr Sheila Baldwin. 'Your death depends on it.'

There is such an impressive string of letters after Dr Baldwin's name I'm amazed it all fits on the business card she offers me. She greets Nigel with a warm smile. Taking a seat at the dining table, she extracts a tan leather writing case containing ivory notepaper and a gold fountain pen from her black briefcase. Cartier no less. Yes, she's the type for a proper pen, I reckon, glancing at the diamond-encrusted rings gracing the third finger of her left hand. The elegant navy suit and cream chiffon top won't be from Marks and Sparks either. Harvey Nichols, I guess. Mid-to-late-forties, of slim build with a feathery caramel mane fluttering around an immaculate, made-up face. Let's hope she's as smart as she looks.

Nigel's on top form today. Cheerful, amusing and displaying zero anxiety. He manages to recount his life story with minimal requirements for me to translate. She records the minutest detail and asks a myriad of questions. Copies of his letter to Dignitas and their response are laid on the table before her, the contents of both analysed and discussed. He emphasises how he's determined to die while he is still happy and smiling.

'What's your opinion of what I plan to do?' he asks, as the meeting draws to a close.

Her response is instant and forthright. 'You're able to discuss your intention for accompanied suicide, in a practical and pragmatic manner. It is clear to me you understand the outcome of such action and there is plenty of evidence to show your capacity to make decisions is not influenced by medication or anxiety.'

We like her.

'Do you agree with the idea of Dignitas? As a doctor?'

'I believe in self-determination,' she says.

That'll do.

Her report pings its arrival on Nigel's email on 21 September. It is forwarded to Dignitas the same day. On 29 September, Nigel receives confirmation that his request is complete, along with an invoice for 3,500 Swiss francs. Once payment is received, his case will be passed to one of their collaborative physicians for consideration. The money is transferred the same day.

And once again, we wait.

26

THE PROVISIONAL GREEN LIGHT

I am a stalker. Albeit a virtual one. If it wasn't for the internet's snooping enabling qualities, I would be forced to camp outside my victim's home, shrouded in hoodie and dark glasses, bearing a rucksack packed with butties and a flask, intent on summoning the courage to confront my prey at the first opportunity. Instead, my stalking gear comprises PJs, pinot, peanuts and a laptop.

I'm poring over a photograph of a family, seated around a table, eating their last meal, hours before the man at the forefront of the image ends his life at Dignitas. They're all smiling. They appear relaxed and happy. This happened last year. Another photograph further down the article shows the family on holiday. Husband and wife and their daughters. I scan the text and, yes, there are names.

Here is a family who recently experienced precisely what we are preparing for. I'm consumed by so many questions. What is Dignitas like? How was her husband at the end? Was he anxious? Did they all accompany him? The kids? How did they travel there? Did she transport his body home? Did a police investigation follow? Should I ask? Dare I? They'll still be grieving. Is it intrusive? I'd hate to upset them. If I'm tactful, maybe? They agreed to be featured in the *DailyMirror*, so they mustn't mind the publicity, right? Their names are there for all to see. Would it hurt?

I start with the wife. She must have a Facebook account. The entire global population has a Facebook account. Shit. She doesn't. The eldest daughter maybe. Bound to be on it. Who isn't on Facebook at twenty-one? I type her name into the search Facebook tab. There she is. Not a great deal on her page. Security-protected no doubt. I must do that with my own. Keep meaning to, never find time. Doesn't matter right now. I'm not interested in rummaging through pics of her family and friends or poking around in her posts. All I want is to send her a message asking if she would connect me with her mum.

What do I say? Having so fiercely guarded our secret, is it wise to reveal our plans to a stranger? I drain and refill my glass. The cursor dillydallies over the Messenger icon. Should I risk it? I gulp the wine. A bit more pinot and I won't care. Setting the glass down, I take a deep breath and make a decision. Ask Nig.

Jeanette's in his room. She'll be tidying up having tucked him in. It shouldn't be awkward for me to wander along the corridor of my own home, slip into Nigel's room and ask Jeanette to leave us for a couple of minutes whilst I discuss something private with my husband. Strange how it seems rude. Stupid I know. Well, he won't be asleep. He'll be on Facebook for hours. I click on his name tag: that profile pic of him captured mid-guffaw and sporting my sunglasses never fails to amuse me. What had happened to provoke such hilarity?

'Get rid of Jeanette. Need a word.'

Moments later, Jeanette wafts by me and into the kitchen. 'His lordship requires a cup of tea.'

'He'll look like a bloody teabag soon,' I say, almost stamping on poor Bodger as I leap to my feet, laptop clutched to my chest.

I shove the article in Nigel's face, point at the daughter and explain my plan.

He recognises the page. 'I've read that,' he says.

Not surprising. If a simpleton took a peek at the search history of my laptop and Nigel's iPad, it would take less than a minute to guess the plan. Dignitas is way up there occupying the top spot, followed by the heart-breaking tales of those who've travelled to die there. Nigel's search history features police interventions, whilst mine focuses on sites covering repatriation of a body. We both read all arguments for and against Dignitas' existence, and similar discussions supporting or denouncing the 'Dignity in Dying' campaign: the majority, well written and persuasive, a few a mere gushing of unsubstantiated opinion.

'Do it,' he says, as Jeanette walks back into the room.

No hesitation over the Messenger tab this time.

'Please forgive this intrusion, I hope you will understand once I explain. I came across the article regarding your father's decision to end his life at Dignitas last year. I offer you and your family my sincere condolences. It must have been a difficult time. My husband has motor neurone disease and he hopes to travel to Dignitas for an accompanied suicide. We're currently awaiting the provisional green light. To speak to someone who has been through this would be extremely helpful. Would you mind asking your mum for her email address so I may contact her? I understand if she would rather I didn't. Thank you for reading this, and once again, I apologise for the intrusion.'

Send. Done. Wait. Stop myself from gawping at Messenger every two minutes. I know I will. She'll have read it already. Young people respond to messages in seconds. She might be on the phone to her mum before I've poured another glass of wine. Look at me, every bit as guilty as Nigel who, impatient as a refugee waiting for passage to freedom, asks 'Has the post arrived?' on a daily basis. Does he imagine I wouldn't tell him? Maybe hide the envelope containing the power to crush him or grant his greatest wish. 'No, why?' I say. 'You waiting for something important?' I close the laptop and vow not to interrogate Messenger until the morning.

It's morning. I peer at Messenger before I unlock the front door for Alison to let herself in. I peep again while boiling the kettle, once I've taken Nigel his cuppa, stare at it the entire time I'm drinking my coffee and fail to resist a sneaky shufty a mere thirteen times while I walk Bodger to the beach and back. Nothing.

On my return, Nigel's parked, as usual, by the island in the kitchen. Alison's busy sorting the wetroom after his shower.

'Heard anything?' he says, grasping the opportunity whilst we're alone to discuss our secret activities.

I kiss his bald head, which smells of Paco Rabanne. He likes to mix things up by demanding the carers apply a different aftershave to his precious bonce every day.

'No. Bugger all.'

'You will,' he says. 'Be patient.'

'Says the epitome of patience.'

He ignores me and points to the article open on his iPad. 'Have a gander at this. "Police investigate wife following husband's death at Dignitas."'

'Aww love,' I say, plonking Bodger on his knee for their morning cuddle.

'Have you brushed him?'

'Yes,' I lie. 'Look, I know you're worried. Try not to be. I've never read anything regarding a prosecution. Have you?'

'No. But –'

'Quick, close it. Alison's coming.'

I shield the iPad from Alison's view. Nigel can't do anything quickly. His hands move like an apprentice welder has grafted the right to his left wrist and the left to his right. I hold my stance until the whoosh of cards dealing a hand of Texas Hold'em releases me.

'Don't lose all your money, buggerlugs.'

Later, the stars conspire to align in such a way the gods are persuaded to post a response on my Messenger tab before my weary eyes pop out. There it is, the mum's email address. 'Welcome to contact at any time.' Now. Now is the time.

My questions surge onto the page. I thank her. Offer my condolences. Express my admiration at hers and her husband's bravery in pursuing a path I still find unimaginable despite imagining nothing else for weeks. I paint a picture of Nigel, his illness and determination to travel to Dignitas.

'Did you ask about prosecution?' says Nigel.

'Yes.'

'Bringing the body back?'

'Of course.'

'Missed anything?'

'No.'

'Go for it.'

Our answers arrive the next day. For once, we are spared the performance of skulking like spies in the shadows, as it's Ellie's shift and once we three are gathered in the kitchen, Nigel refreshed by his shower and soothing daily foot massage underway, I summarise her responses.

'She says Dignitas acted with professionalism throughout.'

'I've found that,' says Nigel.

'She doesn't mention the final day.'

'Not surprised,' says Ellie. 'Not sure I would be happy to share that.'

'Yes. Too painful, perhaps. Anyway, the youngest daughter didn't accompany them as they felt she wasn't old enough, so she stayed with her grandparents.'

'Can't have been easy saying goodbye. Glad I'm coming with you Dad.'

'They flew there, flew back. Paid for the urn to be later transferred to Heathrow and brought home. Organised through Dignitas.'

'No repatriation,' Nigel says.

The disappointment in my voice is evident, as I say, 'No. They were advised against it.'

I had allowed myself to dream this family would show me conveying the body of a loved one home was straightforward. Easy. No, it's far from that. Despite the many websites' promises to take all the stress out of a dreadful situation, to release you from the mind-boggling red tape, to deal with the authorities: police, coroner, consulate, on your behalf, to overcome the language barriers and arrange transport by road or air, it remains a bewildering, time-consuming and distressing process.

Nigel reaches for me. I grasp his hand. 'Julie, I wish you'd give up on the idea.'

'I know you do,' I say, struggling to maintain my composure. 'I can't leave you behind.'

He squeezes my hand with all the strength he has left. 'Let's wait to hear what Dignitas say when, *if*, I'm given the green light.'

My resolve trickles away as I concede. 'OK. Let's do that. It won't be an issue if they don't grant it, will it?' Not one of us considers that likely.

'What about an investigation?' says Ellie, anticipating her dad's next question therefore saving him the effort of speaking.

'A friend of theirs is a lawyer. He spoke with the police when they arrived home from Switzerland. No action taken.'

'Excellent,' says Nigel.

The three of us are silent as I read the email again.

'Anything else?' says Ellie.

'No. That's it. I'll email and thank her for her help.' I head for my laptop wishing her answer regarding repatriation had been different.

...

Adrift in a data-less desert for all of fifteen days, on the afternoon of 14 October 2016, we are buried in the stuff. A bulging A4 envelope thuds onto the mat. The familiar latte colour proclaims its origin. Oh God, it's here. This is it. Nigel's destiny. I make tea, as I do, for no reason at all, and transport both to Nigel's bedroom, where he lies, half-reclined, listening to music on his iPad.

'Ah,' he says, spotting the package and inclining the bed. 'It's here.'

'Yes, indeed it is.' I pop his tea on the bedside table and climb on the bed, clutching the envelope to my chest.

Nigel gawps at me. 'Go on.'

'What? Open it?'

'Go on,' he says.

Apprehensive of what we'll find inside the envelope I mask my fear by making light of it. After all, this doesn't compare to such phenomena as 'My favourite Uni has accepted me.' No, this is, 'Do I die soon, without anxiety and pain? Or do I suffer unspeakable torture for year after agonising year until I die, a shrivelled, tormented shell of the man I used to be?' No. Not the same at all.

I pick at the seal, teasing it open bit by bit. 'Scared?'

'Nah.'

'Liar.'

'Maybe,' he concedes. 'Fuck sake open it.'

'Right, here goes.'

Sliding the contents out of the package, inch by torturous inch, I clutch the pile of papers close to my face. The subject heading leaps from the page. 'Shit.'

'Come on,' says Nigel. 'Let me see.'

'Sorry.' I jump from the bed and hold the letter for him.

'Provisional Green Light

Dear Mr Casson

Please be advised that a medical doctor cooperating with us considers an accompanied suicide to be justified in your case and thus has just given his consent to possibly write the prescription for you. However, the definite decision will only be taken after two personal consultations. You now have the 'provisional green light' for an accompanied suicide in Switzerland.'

'It's happening,' I whisper. Nigel's plan to end his life is progressing. 'It's really happening.'

'How perfect is that?' he says, his face lit by a supernova of joy.

We read on.

'By experience we know that the sole fact of being given the 'provisional green light' for an accompanied suicide in Switzerland might improve your condition, rendering you possibly able to further endure life and even to enjoy it.'

Knowing there is an emergency exit from this world, to pass through at a time of your choosing, has, according to Dignitas, both a life-prolonging and life-enhancing effect. Only a few people granted the provisional green light take up the option. Some 'let go' and die peacefully soon afterwards, whilst others live many more months, years in some cases, with a new and positive attitude, able to bear the unbearable for longer perhaps, as they are in control of their ultimate demise. For Swiss residents, this must be intensely liberating, as Dignitas comes to them. Their accompanied suicide takes place at home. Having made all the preparations, they relax and draw whatever pleasure is possible from each new day, knowing, should things worsen, their release is on hand. But the green light will not prolong Nigel's life, will it? His dying day must be determined whilst he is still able to make the journey. His mood, however, is already vastly improved.

He taps the page with a trembling hand. 'Made my day, that has. I'm so happy.' I swear if he could leap from the bed and prance naked, like a nymph in a forest, he would.

'No shit?' I say, blinded by the sparkle in his eyes.

Like a kid relishing the contents of a glowing school report, he asks, 'What's all the other bumf say?'

'OK let's see. There are personal data sheets to be completed. Easy. Details of you, parents, me, former spouses, kids and so on. A few forms for you to sign giving your instructions. Are you able to sign? A cross or mark of some kind will do, it says.'

'I'll sign.'

'Sure?'

'Certain.'

'OK, and a list of documents they need like passport, birth and marriage certificates, that kind of thing.'

'No problem.'

'No,' I say, reading on. 'Except the certificates must be originals and, what's this mean, "legalised with an Apostille by the British Government?"'

'An apostle?'

'No, apostille.'

'What's that?'

I reach for my phone and Google apostille. 'It's a thing you acquire so official documents are recognised overseas.'

'Bet it's expensive.'

'Bound to be. But required by the Swiss authorities to issue a death certificate.' I drop the pile of papers on the bed. 'Bloody hell, I can't believe we're having this conversation.'

'Come on,' he says. 'Let's complete the forms. Then post them when you walk Bodger.'

'Bit keen aren't we? In a rush, Nig? It says here they need at least three to four weeks to organise an accompanied suicide, and that's after all the documentation is completed. Will you at least give me a chance to pack?'

'Sorry. I'm –'

'Excited?'

'Yes.'

'Dear God.'

The cold practical business of Nigel's accompanied suicide and post-death arrangements occupies the rest of the afternoon. The personal data forms are completed, checked and double-checked. I retreat to a safe zombie-esque state when the whole process of dying and, what happens once dead, decisions are made. In contrast, Nigel couldn't be more delighted to sign the authorisation for

Dignitas to obtain and store the lethal medication in a safe place, until the agreed time of his voluntary death.

'What do you reckon to April?' he says, dragging me from my soothing self-inflicted stupor.

'For what?' I croak.

His smile could not stretch those pale cheeks further. The light could not dance more merrily in those twinkling eyes. 'For dying.'

The pen falls from my hand. 'Bloody hell, Nig.'

'Well, why not? It'll be warmer. And, if it's after the 6th, it will be better for tax.'

I'm awake now. 'For tax? You're planning the day you die around tax advantages?'

'Yep. I'll check with John to be sure.'

I place the papers on the bedside table and prepare to leave. 'I need a drink.'

'Bit early, isn't it?' he says.

'Not for gin. It's never too early for gin.'

'Make mine a whisky,' he calls after me.

It could be the whisky, or more likely the disease causing his hand to tremble as he grips his pen. Despite that, he has no hesitation in scratching an astonishingly legible signature on the instructions regarding medical intervention during the dying phase. There must be no intervention, regardless of how long it takes for him to die. Progress is halted when we reach the form requiring Nigel's instructions on the funeral. Repatriation of the body? Or cremation and return of the urn? I favour repatriation, Nigel, cremation. Yes, I know it's Nigel's body. It's his death, his decision. But I'm his wife. The idea of walking away and leaving him behind rips me apart.

'I'll email Dignitas,' he says.

A reply bounces back within the hour.

'We would not advise a repatriation of the body. This would certainly trigger a police investigation, and would be a hassle for your family.'

That's that. I'm beaten. There's nothing more to say. In fact, I'm unable to speak. Nigel's eyes are teeming with kindness as he raises my hand and brushes it with his lips. Nigel ticks the box for cremation and signs the form. I'm grateful he has the decency not to shout 'Hurray!' Copies are made and safely stored in the red Dignitas folder.

Once finished, Bodger and I hurry Nigel's death plan to the post office.

27

LAST CHRISTMAS

The mouth-watering aroma of sage, onion and chestnut stuffed turkey, swaddled in rosemary and thyme, roasting in the oven, threatens to be overpowered by the intoxicating festive fragrances of cinnamon and cloves, cedar and vanilla, wafting from the flames of Yankee candles and transported by an army of scent-bearing fairies on a quest to saturate the entire flat.

'What's that bloody awful ming?' says Nigel, wheeling into the dining room to escape the fumes.

'Christmas.'

His face scrunches into a pained knot.

'Over the top?'

'Yes. I'm choking to death.'

'Sorry darling.' I resist lighting yet another candle and place the match in its box. 'Getting carried away.'

'Tree looks amazing,' he says.

'Doesn't it though?' I beam, admiring every glittering inch of the spectacular nine-foot creation in the corner. Gold and silver decorations punctuated by the occasional burst of red, arranged,

I would argue, with a level of expertise to match any professional tree decorator. The larger ornaments selected to embellish the lower branches, diminishing in size, not splendour, as the assortment of twinkling trinkets ascend to the sparkling star at the top. Not a single gap remains unenhanced by a pretty bauble and not a branch is bereft of brilliance as hundreds of tiny lights enfold this stunning exhibit in shimmering wonder.

'Paula do it?' he says.

'Yep.'

'Thought so.'

Paula always decorates the tree, sometimes with Ellie's assistance. Both as gifted as Santa's elves in all that is Christmas. My role is limited to lugging the bag bearing the tree from the garage and assembling the thing. Not creatively taxing, more consuming in time and patience, as each individual branch must be slotted into the trunk. I file the decorations by size and colour and pass them to the elf, as required.

'But I did the garlands,' I insist. 'And the table.'

Hidden beneath silken burgundy fabric are two trestle tables placed at one end of our marble dining table, also clothed in burgundy. The table itself seats eight. Today we must accommodate fifteen. Garlands dotted with left-over baubles adorn sequin-studded black velvet central runners. The odd reindeer peeps from behind a bristly fir cone and silver snowmen gather round a Christmas candle. A grandiose five stem candelabra dominates each end of the table and the finest Christmas crackers TK Maxx has to offer are placed on the red and gold chargers of fifteen flawless table settings. The maître d' of London's Ritz would be impressed.

'Right,' says Nigel, seemingly not as impressed as the Ritz's maître d'. His weary expression, tired eyes, encircled by vivid, purple shadows, create a sharp contrast to his pale, sunken cheeks.

'Will you be alright, today?' I ask. 'Do you think you'll cope?'

I'm conscious of how engrossed I've allowed myself to become in the preparations for this special Christmas day, how I relished decorating our home; choosing, buying and wrapping gifts. Paula elf does the wrapping also. How I vacillitated over the menu, before opting for courgette and leek soup, traditional turkey with all the trimmings and yummy old Christmas pud with brandy sauce. How I succeeded in forcing the reality of what we are to face in a few short months from the forefront of my mind, and how critically ill Nigel really is.

'I'll be fine,' he says, wheeling his chair into the sunshine flooded bay. 'I'll sleep now, before the rabble arrive.' He reclines the chair to its extent and is asleep in seconds.

I dash into the kitchen to check on the turkey. Could this be true? A family Christmas? Last year Nigel couldn't tolerate the present opening ceremony, a tradition established once visiting the kids' homes was not an option, given that he couldn't cross the threshold of any of them. I check that everything is ready in the hall, a space the size of most living rooms. Whilst the rest of us flank the walls and surround the pile of gifts in the centre Nigel will be parked at the head, framed by the elaborate stained-glass window, which bears our respective coats of arms, Casson at the top, Murgatroyd below. I'm reminded of both our dads as I look at the window proclaiming their heritage. We lost Dad in 2014, following a series of strokes, and Ron died of heart failure in 2015. Neither would have wanted to witness Nigel ending his life at Dignitas. In previous years, people would be encouraged to leave shortly after the present opening. Not today. For me, today is filled with true gifts. A day for spending precious time as a family. A day for making memories to last a lifetime.

Nigel's decision to go to Dignitas to end his life has freed him from jail. The provisional green light has given him what they said it would – the ability to enjoy the remainder of his life. Once again, laughter echoes throughout our home and Nigel's life is transformed.

The team of carers, still unaware of his plans, are astonished at the change in him. He enjoys his days, instead of enduring them. His appetite has stormed back. After years of picking at soft food, he is requesting and relishing fillet steak. He loves a beer and the occasional whisky and enjoys spending time with family and also the reinstated visits from his golfing mate Gamby, who calls on Friday afternoons without fail, and stays for no more than two hours, at which point Nigel tells him to bugger off. Since the day he made his decision, he has taken not one single Lorazepam. Not one. No longer, when he goes to bed, does he need to swallow three large gulps of morphine. But he still has MND. And he is growing weaker.

I pop the champagne cork from the bottle as the mob descends, chased by four charging miniature schnauzers. Bucks Fizz for Jemma and Amy, as they're but twelve and fourteen and not yet developed a taste for it. Ben and Tom, now fifteen and sixteen and lacking any discernment, down the undiluted stuff like pop. Danny and Daz stack crates of beer and cider in the garage, alongside Tom's non-alcoholic variety and Craig's tonic water. These two non-drinkers doubtless savouring the prospect of telling the rest of us tomorrow how atrociously we behave today. Paula, Ellie and Becky add generous quantities of wine to the already crammed fridge and Charlotte's moderate bottle of gin is broken into. Mum, who never has more than one glass of anything, opts for champers.

'Mmm, smells bloody marvellous in here.'

'When do we eat, I'm starving.'

'We're not having sprouts are we, Grandma? I hate sprouts.'

'Yes, we're having sprouts.'

'Need a hand, Goose?' says Becky. 'Shall I open another bottle of plonk? This one's done the rounds already.'

'Cheers, yes please. Make sure everybody has a drink before we get cracking.'

'Julie, Tom says he's happy to carve the turkey if you like?' offers Paula.

'That'd be helpful. After the pressie opening, please.'

'Lemons?'

'Yes, sliced, in the fridge.'

'Lime?'

'Same.'

'Who wants a beer?'

'Cider for me, mate.'

'Can I do anything, Mum?' says Ellie.

There are no carers coming today, so Nigel will be obliged to make do with me and Ellie. 'Yes please, would you check on your dad in the dining room and take him a beer. Ask him to move into the hall, when he's ready, and remind him he's in charge of the music.'

'Anybody need a top up?'

'Here please.'

'Me too.'

'Cheers.'

Once jackets and hats are dumped in the porch and all glasses filled, the melodious introductory vocals of George Michael's *Last Christmas* emanates from the hall. It stops, unexpectedly. Seconds later, the words 'last Christmas', sung in that incomparable voice, ring out. Stops again. When we hear 'last Christmas' for the third time, the penny drops.

'I don't bloody believe him,' says Craig.

'He's priceless,' says Danny.

'Amazing,' says Daz.

'I'll kill him,' I say.

We file into the hall to find Nigel parked in his customary location, lording it beneath his coat of arms, his eyes flashing with merriment, lips clamped smothering a chortle and, unable to contain it, his head tilts back and that distinctive trumpeting roar bursts unchecked from his mouth. Ellie grabs the bottle of Becks from his hand before his arm jerks and it splashes in his face. Craig, muttering, 'Dad, you're such a twat,' stands beside the chair, should Nigel choke and need help getting up. Becky and I pretend nothing of any signficance is occurring, and usher people into place for the present opening ceremony. Ben and Tom, staring in wonder, down their champagne and grab a beer. Charlotte stands with Jemma and Amy, both biting their lips, while waiting for Grandad to compose himself. Tears well in Paula's eyes and she avoids him altogether. Mum's bewildered, as she hasn't heard a thing and Tom, Daz and Danny survey the scene with appreciative amusement.

'Sorry,' Nigel says, when at last he regains his self-control. 'I couldn't resist.'

Admonished and instructed to play nothing more tragic than *Grandma Got Run over by a Reindeer*, for the rest of the day, we continue with the ceremony. Christmas mornings when the grandchildren dove headfirst into pillowcases bursting with gifts are a thing of the past. Whilst the budget may be the same, the money buys a lot less, and Amy is the solitary grandchild with a respectable pile of parcels at her feet. Designer trainers and tracksuit for Ben; leather jacket, Victoria's Secret underwear and 'anything from New Look' for Jemma; a mere wad of cash for Tom which, despite its presentation inside a Christmas card complete with kisses on the envelope, suggests we don't love him anymore.

We grown ups made a pact, once upon a time, to ease the financial pressure of Christmas and not buy each other presents. After all, there's limited space in the wardrobe for tacky Christmas jumpers and who needs yet more sets of aftershave, bubble bath and body lotion? My persistent cheating means we now exchange thoughtful gifts, combining funds to avoid foisting junk onto one another. Tracy Savage vouchers for the lot of them from me this year. All of us admirers of the local award-winning artist, some adding to our collection of original, dramatic and often humorous artworks inspired by the Yorkshire coastline and landscape, others on the brink of theirs.

...

Had a slice of turkey remained, a solitary pig in a blanket, a morsel of stuffing, a carrot, or a pea, left uneaten, then the dogs would not be so crestfallen. A pitiful handful of sprouts remain at the close of a meal worthy of any chef – including the maître d's mate at the Ritz – whose culinary craft may outstrip my own on 364 days of the year, but not on this day. Nigel, spoon-fed by Ellie, devours hippo portions. His jokes, articulated with agonising care and as unfunny as ever, are listened to with patience and greeted with

polite tittering, much of which is obscured by his own raucous guf-
fawing. Having ceased his tactless tomfoolery, his choice of music
exudes seasonal joy and a sense of celebration.

If it were possible to forget, for a single day, that Nigel has MND,
and no more than a few short months to live, it would be today. As
it is, the combination of rich food, barrel loads of beer and a house-
ful of boisterous revellers, overwhelms him and we are reminded
MND lurks amongst us still.

The merriment stops. His eyelids droop and his face crumples
with fatigue. He surrenders the attempt to speak when the words
won't formulate. His head flops forwards and his whole body
shrinks in on itself, like air expelled from a bag. Accustomed to
spending all day in bed, he is thoroughly washed-out. For him to
withstand a full day's activity is nothing short of miraculous.

'Come on love, let's prepare you for bed.'

'I'll help,' says Ellie.

Nigel mumbles an exhausted, 'Bye, all,' and manages a shaky
wave as we leave the room.

'Night poppet,' says Mum, propelling me fifty-five years back
in time.

'See ya Grandad. It's been cool.'

'Nice one, Nig. Top man.'

Once we're out of the room, people attend to their tasks. The
now familiar pattern of behaviour which has developed during
Nigel's illness kicks in. If there's a job to be done, do it. Don't in-
terfere with what's happening with Nigel, don't be tempted to ask
to help. Stay out of the way, keep quiet and wait. To this end, Paula
and Becky clear the table, fill the dishwasher and feed the dogs.
Danny and Daz offer to refill glasses and everybody else, except

Ben and Tom, who seize the moment to slip away to meet up with mates, retires to the lounge.

'Nig's Christmas Day is over,' I say, on my return. 'He's knackered.'

'He's astounding,' says Mum.

'Isn't he? A one off. I'm so proud of him.'

'Is he asleep?' says Craig.

'No, Ellie's making him a cuppa before he settles down. He won't be long.'

'OK if we nip and say goodbye? We'll be off soon.'

'Of course, go ahead.'

Craig and his family pop to see Nigel. Mum accepts the offer of a lift home, and before the wrangling about teams for Trivial Pursuit gets underway, Nigel is snoozing like Rip Van Winkle.

The last ever Christmas we will spend with Nigel is over.

28

THE RECCE

It's time to break out the 'deal with it later box' from its prison in the bit drawer inside my head, and release that nagging question: how do we transport Nigel from Scarborough to Zurich?

The mission is underway. Fly. Obviously. Fast. Easy. Ah, no. Not easy at all. All of two seconds to quash that plan. Wheelchair users cannot travel in their own chairs: the wheelchair is stored in the hold. Users are transferred to a compact chair which transports them onto the plane before being transferred to a seat. Not a chance. Superman and his heroic mates would struggle to lift him from his customised carriage without a hoist. Manhandling him would prompt a panic attack, his legs would spasm, he'd slip into donkey birthing mode and terrify the other passengers, and anyway, there's no way he has sufficient muscle tone to occupy a normal seat. He'd flop like a rag doll with all its stuffing ripped out.

'What about a chartering a private jet?' says Nigel.

'Bloody hell, Rockefeller. Splashing some cash around, aren't we?' It would, however, resolve the problem of the other passengers.

'Well, it's my last holiday, isn't it?'

'Holiday?'

'Yes. An adventure,' he cries. 'Five go to Zurich.'

'Nig, you're unbelievable. You'd render Enid Blyton lost for words.'

OK, let's have a crack at that. After all, money makes anything possible, so they say. I won't pretend I don't relish the idea of jetting across the skies like royalty, and I pursue this tantalising prospect with enthusiasm bordering on inappropriate. As is always the case, it doesn't take long for practicalities to destroy dreams.

How expensive would it be, for discretion not to be an issue? Where staff are so professional not a single brow is raised when a terminally ill and physically disabled passenger requests a one-way flight to Zurich? Any chance of hitching a lift in a Chinook, Daz? He knows a couple of ex-RAF pilots who work for private jet companies, so he has a word. They have no need to meet Nigel to guess what we're up to. No, is the answer.

It doesn't signify anyway. Money can't buy everything, as it happens. Mark Zuckerberg's fortune and an army of personnel as close-lipped as corpses could not make it possible for Nigel to travel in a seat on an aeroplane. For a minute, I toy with the idea of an air ambulance, until a modicum of research convinces me the accompanying medical staff would oppose the reason for our journey and decline to fly us.

We five who will not go to Zurich in a private jet are gathered in the lounge for one of our clandestine get-togethers. Craig is the only one of us not disappointed by the discarded option of flying. Not a keen flyer, he prefers to plot flight paths via an app from the safety of the ground, and to explore the intricate arteries of his substantial ordnance survey map collection, on foot.

'Driving?' he says.

'You don't mean the Berlingo?' I say, horrified. 'Bit of a come down from a private jet.'

'It'd be a laugh,' says Nigel, chortling.

He's joking. Got to be. I glare at him, regardless.

'No, it's too small. An adapted Transit van maybe? You know, like the accessible taxis.'

'Who'd do the driving?' says Ellie. 'You?'

'Or hire a taxi?' I interject. That is a joke.

'No chance,' says Craig, ignoring me. I'm not driving all that way with my back. I'll be wrecked by the time we reach Staxton. Anyway, you two have driven across Europe loads of times.'

'Train?' says Becky, lobbing an alternative into the pot.

I like that. 'Much better idea.' I've always liked trains. Civilised way to travel. First Class all the way.

Four faces turn to Nigel. He concurs.

Plan B is born. The train it is.

'We should do a recce,' says Becky.

Not for nothing has she risen swiftly to the rank of Sergeant. A meticulous organiser who assesses the risks, expects the unexpected, tests each component of the plan and stands ready with options should anything fall apart.

'Great idea. You and Mum do the recce. I need Ellie here.'

'Is a recce necessary?' says Ellie, who rarely appreciates the degree of her sister's preparation, preferring instead to tackle whatever confronts her, head on. On this occasion, however, she concedes before Becky launches a passionate defence of her recce. 'Maybe you're right. And you might as well check out the hotel's disabled facilities while you're there.'

'Is the hotel sorted?' says Craig.

'Not quite. I have a shortlist of one. Your dad's still getting over the price.'

'We'll check it out. Makes sense.'

...

Armed with specially commissioned notebook and pen, iPad for recording data and taking photographs, sturdy tape measure with which to establish the width of doorways, aisles, wheelchair spaces and alleys between Scarborough and Zurich, Becky and I pound Scarborough's railway station like representatives from Disabled UK. It's adequate. Do-able. We consider the idea of one of us travelling in a wheelchair for the sake of realism then dismiss it as images of me behaving like Matt Lucas's Andy in *Little Britain*, gambolling up and down platforms pirouette inside my head. We record the dimensions of Nigel's larger than average custom-made chair instead, and the phone numbers and locations of assistance staff in all connecting stations from here to Zurich.

Once aboard and settled in the deserted First-Class carriage which smells of new leather and the lingering perfume of a disembarked passenger, we update the checklist. Or is it a spreadsheet? Becky's in charge of admin. I contribute by saying, 'Tick'. Tape measure ready for action. Will the chair fit? Tick. Wheelchair space? Tick. Enough? Tick. Toilet? Yes, the modern type with a sliding door. Measure the space. Yes, Nigel's chair should make it inside if we need to empty his catheter bag in private. Unlikely as it's a mere ten minutes into the journey. I afford it a tick for completeness. We're nothing if not thorough. That's it. So far so good. We relax. Isn't it brilliant when things work out? We might even enjoy the journey.

We get as far as York. Were it not for the human requirement to use the toilet, travelling with a severely disabled person would be no problem at all. Only specialist 'Changing Places' toilets equipped with ceiling hoist and adult changing area are suitable for Nigel and, whilst it may be part of its improvement plan, York has no such facility and therefore receives the first 'X' of the day. King's Cross Station has, however, so if Nigel needs the loo between Scarborough and Zurich, it's King's Cross or nowhere.

Pretending our legs are wheels, we avoid the stairs to the bridge over which I have wobbled, following many a lunch in York, and take the lift to the disabled access corridor which runs beneath the tracks. I resolve to follow this route more often. It's nowhere near as crowded and, if one has had one or two pinots, a lot less precarious. Must mention it to Mel. It would save her from tumbling down those steps again.

All is well. Becky and I bubble with positivity as our Grand Central connecting train to King's Cross hurtles onto the platform a minute earlier than scheduled. The stifled murmurings of London-bound commuters pervade our allotted First-Class carriage along with the obnoxious combined odours of coffee and old men's heads, both of which cling to the scratchy palette of all shades brown, shabbier than chic seats.

'Bit of an old rattler this, isn't it?' I say, placing my bag in the rack overhead.

'There's no wheelchair space either,' says Becky, not inclined to forget the objectives of our operation.

'You're right. Maybe there's one in a different carriage.'

'You didn't ask when you booked, Goose?' she says, every inch the Sergeant as she peers at me from beneath one raised eyebrow. I know the expression, the disappointed face which screams: 'Can you do nothing right?' It's exactly like mine.

'I booked online. Assumed ....'

The second eyebrow raises to join the first.

'OK, I know, never assume and all that. I'll find out.'

I flee from the carriage in search of absolution and a wheelchair space, careful not to look back, lest I'm transformed into a pillar of salt.

Four carriages on, the amiable ticket collector, apologises, in a soft Geordie accent 'Eee, sorry, pet. If there is one, it's at the far end of the train. Chances are, pet, you need Grand Central's other type of train, like.'

Brilliant. I've booked the wrong type of train. Why more than one type? Instead of a wrong and a right type, why not two right types? Oh dear, this will bugger up Becky's spreadsheet good and proper.

I slink back to my seat.

'Well?' says Becky as I slide beside her.

'Lesson one,' I say. 'Book a Virgin train.'

Those eyebrows raise again.

'No wheelchair spaces on this train.'

'Indeed,' she says, switching on her iPad, no doubt intending to update the spreadsheet with the instruction: under no circumstances allow Mum to book the trains.

'However,' I continue, reaching into the package I collected from the buffet car on the way back to my seat. 'They do have wine.'

...

The Changing Places toilet at King's Cross station is next to platform nine. We know this as we studied the map on the iPad. Determined to be thorough, we walk the route anyway. As we weave our way through the concourse, slipping niftily by M & S and Boots, skirting the crowds outside Costa, dodging the ankle-smashing luggage dragged along by harried travellers, the first tentacle of unease pricks at my temple.

'Is this a station or a shopping centre?'

'Pretty much both,' says Becky. 'You OK?'

'I am. Not sure your dad will be.'

You expect London's stations to be bustling. But Nigel, who's unable to tolerate more than two guests at a time, will panic when confronted by this clamour of shifting bodies. His chair couldn't duck the crowds. He'd barge through the masses like a rampant bull, trampling a few on his way.

'We'll need a skip load of Lorazepam to keep your dad calm. Not to mention me.'

We stop to check the information signs. Platform nine over there. Exit to St Pancras this way. On it.

'You know,' says Becky as we plough on through the melee. 'We should employ passenger assistance staff more effectively. They'll do more than provide the ramp for transferring Dad on and off the train. They'll guide him through the station.'

I gaze with admiration into my daughter's intelligent nutmeg brown eyes.

'You're not bad at this, are you? Add that to the spreadsheet.'

...

If we could board the Eurostar in Scarborough and alight in Zurich, there would be no need for a recce. Wheelchair users travel Standard Premier, or Business Premier, for the price of Standard Class. We opt for Business Premier, which means we'll take advantage of a speedy check in, luxuriate in the private lounge prior to departure, and parktake of some light refreshment. Once on the train we discover there is ample space for Nigel's chair, with a table upon which complimentary meals and drinks are served. All within easy reach of a toilet which, whilst not as perfect as 'Changing Places', is adequately proportioned for the discreet emptying of a catheter bag. Bliss. Bliss. Bliss.

Then. Paris.

We emerge from the Gare du Nord to be spewed into the gaping mouth of Hell. A frenetic multitude of darting humanity gushes around us like goblins on crack. I'm not sure if they are entering or departing from the station as they swirl this way and that, as agitated as if Old Nick had lit a match to their undies.

'*Merde,*' I murmur.

'Fuck,' says Becky.

We have ninety minutes to cross the city to reach the Gare de Lyon, where we make our connection to Zurich. The wheel-chair-accessible taxi, booked for precisely that reason, is nowhere in sight. I reach for my phone and dial the company while digging what little French I can remember from the depths of my memory. My French improves when I'm drunk, and I'm far from that. I say my name and babble something along the lines of, '*Reserve un taxi. Gare du Nord. Ce n'est pas ici.*'

'*Oui, il est en route. Quinze minutes.*'

'It'll be fifteen minutes.'

'Not looking too clever, is it?' says Becky. She checks her watch. Chews at her bottom lip.

'No. Maybe this mode of travel is not the best.'

It's twenty minutes, in fact, before the taxi arrives and he's determined to waste the remaining seventy as he inches through the bedlam that is Paris. When the vast, palatial façade of the Gare de Lyon comes into view, we have a paltry thirty minutes before our

Zurich train leaves. The snake of taxis coiling to the drop-off point stretches for 500 metres. We'll never make it.

'We'd better run,' says Becky.

I pay the driver. We leap from the taxi and race towards the station, tackling the many steps leading to the concourse, two at a time. This is, of course, impossible for Nigel. The magnificent arched entrance beckons and the elegant clock tower ticks as if to remind us how little time we have. There'll be no time to appreciate the grandeur of this sprawling, majestic building. Not for us a relaxing drink in the Big Ben Bar, or the opportunity to take advantage of the Salon Grand Voyageur, despite having tickets to do so. Becky's making excellent progress. I sprint behind as speedily as my bouncing bag and lungs will allow. Not far now. Almost there. A few more strides. At last. We're in.

If the Gare du Nord delivered us to the mouth of Hell, the Gare de Lyon propels us, spiralling past the 'Nine Circles' of Dante's *Inferno*, to the nucleus of Satan's living room.

'*Merde,*' murmurs Becky.

'Fuck,' I say.

Compared to this, King's Cross station is a dreamy, solitary wander through meadows of Wordsworth's hosts of golden daffodils. This station provides a gateway to the whole of Europe. At its core, throngs of aggravated people dart in all directions, zigzagging like swarms of jostling ants through the concourse in search of their departure point. Penetrating cries of '*Allez! Allez!*' and '*Non, par ici!*' battle with insistent calls to '*Komm, schnell!*' 'Hurry. This way!' Clamorous announcements echo-like warnings from the tannoy system, clashing with the pulsating clatter of thousands of luggage wheels. I'm struck by a disturbing sense of urgency. An aura of repressed panic. This is what it must be like to flee from a war zone.

Becky and I stand hypnotised amid this pandemonium and come to the same conclusion. This is beyond Nigel. He can't do this.

'It's not happening,' I say.

'Not a chance. But let's not give up yet,' says Becky. 'There's still the hotel to check out.'

There is no need for me to retrieve the sturdy tape measure from my bag when we board the LGV Lyria train to Zurich, to know with complete certainty, Nigel's chair would struggle to access the carriage. The gap itself is obstructed by luggage which, if removed, would make no difference as the wheelchair space itself is inadequate.

'Is this First Class?' says Becky, wrinkling her nose in disdain as we take our seats.

'Supposed to be. Not impressed?'

'No. We're accustomed to better quality than this, Mama Goose.'

'You're spoilt by Eurostar. Maybe I should've booked Business Class. A champagne-drenched meal is served in that category.'

The carriage is not unlike that of the Grand Central, favouring every shade of drab and drabber on the spectrum. However, it's comfortable and clean. We're not sharing a table seat with strangers, and we'll be in Zurich in a little more than four hours.

'So long as they serve wine,' she says, eyeing the food and drink menu tucked in the seat pocket in front of us.

As if reading her mind, the carriage door opens and the service trolley trundles in, guided by a smartly attired attendant who is so petite she does well to manoeuvre the bulky contraption. A navy tunic, edged with crimson, is harmonised by a crimson cravat. Matching scrunchie binding a sweeping honeysuckle blonde ponytail, coordinated painted fingernails and vivid lipstick, combine with her dazzling smile to eclipse the dreariness of our surroundings.

'*Bonjour mesdames,*' she beams.

Vivienne, as her name badge indicates, appears to be one of those rare people who loves her job.

'*Bonjour,*' we say in unison. One word is sufficient for her to recognise our Englishness. She switches languages effortlessly.

'Would you like to order?'

'White wine, please.'

'A sandwich?'

We order ham and cheese.

She places glasses on our tables and rummages in the trolley for the wine. 'Are you travelling with us all the way to Zurich?'

'Yes,' we say.

'Your first visit?'

'Yes.'

We clutch the bottles of pinot grigio. 'Thank you.'

'Mother and daughter?' she continues.

Oh dear. More questions. 'Yes.' Please give us the sandwiches.

Undeterred by our monosyllabic responses, this amiable attendant persists.

'Holiday?' she says. 'Zurich is so beautiful.'

'Er –' I stutter.

'A short break,' says Becky. A markedly swifter thinker than me.

'Have a wonderful time,' she says, handing over the sandwiches before they're stale. 'Enjoy my city.'

I wait until Vivienne has moved further down the carriage before speaking. 'That was awkward.'

'Wasn't it? She's lovely. Felt a bit rude.'

'I know what you mean. We can hardly tell her the truth, though. Anyway, we won't bump into her again, so it doesn't matter.'

It's approaching midnight when our pre-arranged car delivers us to the Dolder Grand Hotel, Zurich's top address since 1899. Had it not been so late, we might have taken the time to appreciate the magnificence of this outstanding hotel, perched 200 metres above Zurich's city centre, boasting spectacular views of the city, the lake and the Alps. We must trust the website's blurb regarding this fairy tale castle, until we judge for ourselves in the morning. The resplendent entrance lobby is doubtless more predisposed to receiving royalty and A-list celebrities than two travel-weary Yorkshire lasses on a recce. Still, our money is as good as anybody's, and business awaits.

When booking, I had informed the hotel's 'one of a kind' concierge service of our intention to return in April, with my disabled husband, and the purpose of this trip was to inspect their disabled facilities. The receptionist assures us this is arranged for the morning. He goes on to tell us this is the one night of the year when the hotel checks its entire electrical circuits, and all the lights will be switched off between 0100 and 0600 hours as guests are expected to be asleep. Also, if we require some refreshments, please order now before the kitchen is shut down.

He must be joking. 'Pardon?' He explains again. He's not joking.

'Are they changing all the light bulbs, or what?' says Becky.

We bathe by candlelight and navigate our luxurious room illuminated by the torches on our phones and the twinkling panorama provided courtesy of Zurich's city centre.

The following morning, we are escorted throughout the hotel by one of those incomparable concierges. Behaving like a spoilt celebrity, I dismiss the first two rooms offering disabled facilities.

Tape measure in hand, we establish the adequacy of the facility's dimensions like a couple of ladies in waiting requiring the housing of the entire collection of Imelda Marcos's shoes. Sorry, insufficient space. We must also dine in the room, Nigel won't be spoonfed in public. No, this won't do either. Needs a larger shower area. He'd never fit into this toilet space. Insufficient grab rails. We need a suite for a disabled guest with an adjoining room providing easy access for the girls. A third room is required for Craig. All on the same floor. Next to each other if possible. When at last our needs are met, the appropriate room numbers are recorded. Tick.

I'm convinced the 'ask us anything' concierge service wishes I would please stop asking anything at all, when I enquire about the provision of a mobile hoist and shower chair. His blank expression confirms I've blown his mind. Could be a language issue of course, but I suspect the equipment needs of disabled people are a mystery to him.

'No problem. I'll email a list of what we require, with photographs, once we're home.'

'Thank you, Madam, that would be excellent.'

Our car arrives to whisk us to the station before we've had a chance to swallow a mouthful of breakfast. Here we go again. As we descend the hill, a glance behind confirms this exclusive hotel is indeed a fairytale castle, within whose towering spires the tragic Rapunzel could cheerfully dwell.

This is Zurich and therefore our train is precisely on time. The carriage is the same one from which we disembarked a mere eleven hours ago. Within thirty minutes of our departure, the door slides open to admit the tea and coffee trolley.

'Don't look now, Goose,' says Becky.

I look. 'Shit.' Vivienne.

Her radiance vanishes as she reaches our seats. 'Ladies? Back so soon?'

'Er –' I mutter once more. It would seem this is all I'm capable of when confronted with this attendant.

'Change of plan,' lies Becky with impressive ease. 'We'll come back another time.'

'Shame,' says Vivienne, as she serves our coffee and moves on. I swear she's affronted by our failure to allow Zurich the chance to charm us.

'I think we've upset her,' I say. 'Although you did tell her we were here for a short break.'

'Yes, but not how short.'

I'm convinced we must have offended Vivienne when, a couple of hours later, the trolley bearing drinks and snacks reappears without her. She is replaced by a middle-aged giant of a bloke, whose rosacea complexion and clumps of hair sprouting from his ears convey the impression of a man who doubles as a scarecrow. We decline further refreshments in favour of the Eurostar.

Once cocooned within the opulent haven of the Eurostar, having enjoyed a delectable lunch, we consult our records and review the spreadsheet.

'What could we do differently?' I ask.

'Apart from making sure there's wheelchair space on the train from York to London?' says my Sergeant daughter.

'OK. Point taken.'

'Also, book passenger assistance in advance at every station and connection.'

'If the taxi is late in Paris, like yesterday and we miss the connection, then what?'

'We book earlier trains, with longer connecting gaps, giving us loads of wriggle room.'

'You're amazing at this.'

'I know. It's my job.'

I lean back in my seat. 'Is it still do-able? With those amendments?'

Becky takes a long sip of her wine and ponders the spreadsheet before her.

'No,' she says, at last. 'There are too many moving parts. A late train or a last-minute replacement train, which might lack wheel-chair space, the potential absence of a passenger assistance team member, the time it takes for a taxi to reach the drop off point at the Gare de Lyon, the lack of space on the Paris to Zurich train, the length the day would need to be to take all that into account, and the overall lack of toilet facilities. One hiccup and Dad's stuffed.'

'Long list.'

'Plus, there are other major things outside our control.'

'Like?'

'The crowds,' she says. 'And Dad.'

Although we've known in our hearts since we alighted at King's Cross, we finally admit defeat. The decision is made. We're not travelling by train.

We slump, dejected, in our seats. Notebook and iPad, redundant, are placed in our respective bags. Perhaps it was always unrealistic to hope we could travel over 800 miles with a profoundly ill, disabled man, on public transport. Especially when the overriding problem of his condition is the public.

Before we contemplate alternative means of travel within Nigel's capability, my phone rings. Ellie. FaceTime.

'Hi,' we say, our heads pressed together to fit the screen.

Ellie stands behind Nigel, her chin resting on his shoulder as they both grin into the phone.

'How you doing?' says Ellie.

'Could be better,' I reply.

'Too many moving parts,' adds Becky. 'Dad can't do it.'

'Thought so when you mentioned the crowds at King's Cross,' says Ellie, a wide grin on her face. Hardly an appropriate countenance when things are progressing so dismally.

Nigel's faltering voice interrupts the chatter. 'We could have saved you the trouble,' he croaks. 'Not to mention money.'

'What do you mean?'

Smug now, Ellie says, 'Dad's found a massive motorhome for hire. Equipped for disabled use, with ramp, profiling bed, ceiling hoist and toilet.'

'You're kidding?'

'No, I'm not. It's perfect.'

'Bloody hell,' says Becky. 'We needn't have bothered.'

'My thoughts exactly,' says Ellie. 'Recce my arse.'

'Fuck off,' Becky counters.

Their sparkling faces assure me this is sisterly banter.

'No, wait a minute,' I insist. 'At least we've checked out the hotel. Even you thought that was a sensible idea.'

'Fair one,' says Ellie. 'Now hurry home you two and we'll tell you all about it.'

We end the call and, once again, Becky and I sink into our seats. I don't know whether to be delighted or pissed off. Has this been a complete waste of time?

When Becky says, 'It's sorted. Just like that. Can you credit it?' I reach for her hand. 'Don't be disheartened, Bex. The recce was a sensible move. We've learned a lot.'

'Yes, Goose, we have. Not to do it again.'

'Which was the whole point of it, after all.'

'True enough,' she says, appeased.

As I open my mouth to say, 'We should celebrate,' I marvel at the notion that the means of transporting Nigel to his death could be considered grounds for celebration.

'Wine?' she says.

'No. Let's make it champagne.'

29

APPOINTMENT WITH DEATH

The lads are back. The 2017 Six Nations Rugby Championship kicks off today, and Graham, Bruce and Tom are joining Nigel for some intense blokey activity, involving beer and an abundance of hearty banter. Danny and Daz, not lured by their favoured football fixtures today, choose to join us for this superior sporting revelry.

Dressed in his red British Lions rugby shirt, Nigel awaits his guests in the lounge.

I won't ask how he'll cope. No need. Not since the god of the green light showed up and performed its miracle, at which point the terrors were expelled from his mind and the healing power of control restored to his life. Here he is, reclined, dude-like, in his chair, iPad set to operate the TV, bottle of Becks on the side table, twenty quid ready for the inevitable wager, legs crossed casually at the ankle, cheeks flushed with a grin anticipating a contest full of delights. Two matches: Scotland v Ireland, England v France. The preamble: half time; concluding analysis; more preamble; another half time; yet more analysis. Food and booze slotted in and among.

I survey the platter of tuna mayo, ham and cheddar and beef and red onion sandwiches.

'Do we need more?'

'No,' says my Six Nations catering partner, Paula. 'We've mini pizzas as well, don't forget.'

'OK. But Bruce can eat for England. And, for a skinny one, Daz shifts a cartload of grub.'

I cut pork pies into quarters and add them to the buffet. The food selected so Nigel can feed himself, rather than for its gastronomic qualities. Paula will doubtless take up the challenge of producing a more exacting menu in the coming weeks, but this initial offering will suffice. It's man food. They're men. Sorted.

The guests arrive. Bruce, a chain-smoking heavy drinker who carries as much charm as he does weight, plonks eighteen cans of Special Brew on the island in the kitchen.

'Bloody hell, will you have enough?' I ask.

'They're to accommodate next week's merriment also, my good woman,' he says. Considering Bruce is a bear of man, he speaks like he's dropped from the pages of a Jane Austen novel. 'Not a drinking man I, as you know. If you hear anything to the contrary, 'tis a vicious rumour.'

'Indeed.'

'Ladies, this is for you,' says Graham, handing us a quality Italian pinot grigio before opening a can of San Miguel. 'You do like it. You drank plenty at the pub.' Ah, the delightful Indigo Alley. Our dash to after-work pub. Graham and Irene sold it a few years since, planning to spend large chunks of their retirement at their apartment in Spain. Fate, however, has a knack of shattering dreams, and cancer stole Irene's future soon afterwards.

Graham and Bruce, unaware of Nigel's plans, won't appreciate how precious the time spent with Nigel will be over the forthcoming weeks. Unfair as we think it is to exclude them from the secret, it is for Nigel to determine in whom he confides, and when. There is a celebratory air as the sporting enthusiasts take their seats and the temperate Tom dismisses his usual non-alcoholic beverage, in favour of a Peroni.

'Who's your money on, estimable host?' says Bruce.

'Ireland to beat Scotland,' says Nigel.

'Sassenach!' says Graham, a Scot.

'England to beat France in the second match.'

'Scotland will prevail. Mark my words.'

'It'll be close, I reckon.'

'I'm betting France.'

'Not a chance.'

'England are a strong team. I reckon they could win the championship.'

Paula and I whet appetites with half the sandwiches and pork pies, promise to keep supplies coming throughout the day's entertainment, and head for the kitchen to sample the fine Italian pinot.

...

Whilst I focus on organising Nigel's social diary, Nigel is consumed with organising his death.

Olivia's recent medical report is attached to Nigel's second letter requesting an accompanied suicide, and both are placed in the envelope. The letter doesn't differ much from the one written back in August. It stresses how his condition has deteriorated further, how he spends most of his day in bed and how he is unable to attend to any personal needs. The vital components, required by Dignitas, apart from the need for up-to-date correspondence, are that Nigel still wishes to proceed, his decision is not influenced by medication, and he is still judged to be terminally ill. Yes. Both documents should meet Dignitas's final requirements. I place copies in the file next to the section bearing duplicates of certificates, complete with apostille, already in the post. Yet shedloads of jobs remain.

'My contact person is asking what to do with the urn,' says Nigel.

He or she who has no name, a person who closes all emails from Dignitas with 'your contact person,' is unarguably efficient. Responses to Nigel's emails arrive the same day, the English and grammar are faultless, and Nigel is encouraged to ask as many questions as he wishes. Conveyed in as casual a manner as the proposed despatch of a knitted jumper, our contact person informs us our illustrious Royal Mail no longer allows urns to be forwarded by post. We, are therefore, left with two options: enlist the services of a British undertaker, contact name, address, phone number and email provided below, who will, for a fee, arrange airfreight to the UK and deliver to any address; or a designated person collects the urn from the crematorium in Zurich or Dignitas's office, approximately ten days after the demise.

'Bit expensive,' says Nigel, eyeing the funeral director's fee.

'Are you for real?'

He grins. 'Leave me there, for all I care. Chuck me in a wheelie bin.'

People say things like this all the time. They don't mean it. And if he does, I'm not standing for it. Still struggling with the prospect of leaving his body behind, abandoning his ashes is not an option.

'Sod off, Nig. It's a lot bloody cheaper than carting your body back. I'm not going back to Switzerland for your urn and I'm not leaving you there. Decision made.'

Choosing not to engage in this battle, he submits. 'OK, you win.'

Nigel's fondness for money is legendary. As a child he would relieve gas meters of the stuff all the time. He would also, at every opportunity, dip into his dad's carelessly discarded wallet, which bulged with takings from the gambling club. On reaching eleven, and weary of beatings, his criminal career came to an end. Work, honest, endless work proved the solitary option and in this, he excelled. He's no penny pincher, nor is he reckless. He never exploits others and rarely is he ripped off. His inherent sense of fairness may well explain his success in business. Nonetheless, if he considers the price of something to be less than reasonable, he is adamant in his refusal to pay it.

The next pressing item on Nigel's dying agenda is the date.

'I'm thinking back end of April,' he says.

I grab the calendar from its nail on the pantry door. The calendar, Mum's annual creation, featuring photographs of the family, is dominated this year by images of her eightieth birthday bash. Captured looking years short of eighty, Mum, surrounded by four of her grandchildren, exudes happiness as she beams at the camera. Memories depicting enjoyable times: Mum, perched on Nigel's knee, Jemma and Amy, hugging one another, Becky, chilling on a beach, me and Jez, locked in earnest conversation, Craig, standing on his head, Tom, chuckling in a corner. Pictures taken long before Dignitas became part of our lives. Who amongst us could predict back then, what we are facing now?

I flick forward to April. Two pages. That's all it is. A matter of weeks.

We pour over the dates as though planning a spring picnic in the park. We'll be praying for fine weather next. Must be here for the Casson Shield on the 9th. Nigel intends to present his prize one last time. We're into Easter already. My head near explodes when I contemplate the journey at any time, but we must avoid travelling on a Bank Holiday.

'Let's aim to arrive at the hotel by Sunday 23rd,' he suggests.

'Remember we've to see the doctor two days on the trot.'

'Which leads us to the 26th.'

'Or maybe,' he says, 'the 25th, if he visits Sunday night and again on Monday.'

'True. In a rush, are we?' That date rings a bell. Why can't I place it?

A cheeky grin settles on his face. 'Sooner the better. Get it over with.'

I remember. 'You do know 25 April is Ellie and Danny's wedding anniversary, don't you?'

'Is it?'

'Yes.'

He leaves it in the hands of providence. 'Never mind. Let's see what Dignitas arranges with the doctor. I'll email the dates now.'

'Mm hum.' I stare at the calendar. 25th? 26th? Does it matter? By the 27th Nigel will be dead. I stare until the numbers blur to a splodge. Nigel traps a treacherous tear as it trickles down my cheek.

'Julie,' he murmurs. 'Come on now.'

I drop the calendar on the bed. 'Sorry,' I sniff.

...

Nigel's contact person is slacking. It's taken all of twenty-four hours to respond. '25 April confirmed,' the subject states. I send the message to the printer while scanning the text. Oh, this could be interesting. Thank God it's Ellie's shift. This row won't wait.

Shower completed; Ellie prepares to hoist Nigel back into bed.

'You have a date,' I announce, marching into the bedroom, brandishing the email aloft.

Both heads spin towards me. Ellie takes her hand off the button. Nigel dangles mid-air.

'When?'

'Let him down,' I say. 'Make him comfortable.'

'When?' says Nigel, as Ellie completes the manoeuvre and plumps his pillows. 'Come on.'

I hold their attention. '25 April.'

'Ha ha.' Nigel honks. 'Brilliant.'

'Wait a minute, twenty-fifth?' says Ellie, glaring beneath a crumpled brow. She shoots Nigel a piercing glance and glowers at me with a distinct dash of the amateur dramatics.

''Fraid so, darling. I did warn him.'

'Humph! Cheers Dad,' she says, adopting a combatant's stance, hands on hips and jutting chin. 'Now my wedding anniversary will be forever overshadowed by your death-versary.'

'Funny. I like that. "Death-versary." It'll help you remember it. Danny won't bollock you for forgetting a card.'

Ellie's fleeting grimace dissolves in a breath. She waves her arms, dismissing the matter. 'Nah, it's OK. I'm not serious. We don't bother with all that shite.'

'There you are. Your mum will stop tutting at me, now.'

I dither a moment, before adding, 'There's more.'

'What a day this is,' says Ellie.

'Let's hear it.' says Nigel.

I take a deep breath. 'The doctor says it's possible to meet you at the Dolder Grand on the Sunday and Monday.'

'Great,' says Nigel.

'Better book the hotel,' says Ellie.

'But,' I continue.

'But what?' says Nigel.

Another deep breath. 'But the hotel's out of his area, so, there's a slight additional charge.'

The silence stretches on and on.

'How slight?' says Nigel.

I can't voice the amount, so I close his hand around the paper and let him read the mail himself. Ellie slots his glasses on his face. He inclines the bed and reads. Slowly. His expression impassive as he absorbs the text.

'Fuck that!'

'Come on Nig,' I venture.

'Two grand! Not a fucking chance.'

'Wow. That's a lot,' says Ellie.

My eyes flash danger.

'Look Nig, we're talking Swiss francs, not pounds, and it includes an extra five hundred because he's coming on a Sunday, so, that's to pay for regardless, on top of the standard fee.'

The contact person must have gained some insight into Nigel's personality, as he or she lists four alternative hotels, close to the doctor's surgery, where the ransom is not so extortionate. The surgery itself is out of the question, given its inaccessibility to wheelchair users. I'm inclined to express my outrage at this shocking exclusion, however, now is not the time.

'Will you at least discuss it?'

'No,' he barks.

'Please.'

'No.'

To continue the argument would be fruitless. He signals for the NIPPY. Ellie applies the nose pillow to his nostrils, adjusts the strap around his head and switches on the ventilator. Leaning into the pillow he closes his eyes. An hour should do it. He'll calm down, though he still won't be in a mood to discuss this.

I brush my lips on his brow. 'Relax. Leave it with me. Don't worry.'

Absorbed in my laptop, I analyse the information and Google the driving time to the four alternative hotels from the Dolder Grand. Between twelve and sixteen minutes. Disabled facilities and wheelchair accessible taxi companies, next.

OK, let's consider how this could play out. Let's say it will take approximately twenty-four hours travelling time, in the motorhome, to drive from Scarborough to Zurich. Assuming all goes well. Will Nigel be exhausted? Er, who am I kidding? He'll be near dead with fatigue. And he won't be alone. We all will. So, then what? Unpack? Bite to eat? Relax? Shower? Settle down for a snooze? No, stupid idea, Julie. Let's jump in a taxi and head for an unfamiliar city centre. Be sure to give ourselves plenty of time, arrive at the rendezvous hotel well before the doctor. Wait. Meet the doctor. How will we know him? White carnation? Maybe he'll be wielding a bloody brolly over his head? Proceed with what will be the most critical and private medical exchange of Nigel's entire life – in a public place. Once done, await another taxi. Return to the Dolder Grand. Repeat the entire process the following day. All this, instead of the doctor visiting Nigel, in our hotel room.

No, no, no. Nigel, you must not do this. You can't. And for what? To save a few quid? A mere five hundred francs? This is the guy who's given you the provisional green light. Your discussion with this doctor will determine if the green light is confirmed. How crucial could this be? Dear God, you couldn't invent a more life and death scenario. Why, of all things would you choose to squeeze the budget on that? No way should you impose a limit on this vital aspect of your whole Dignitas plan.

Ellie appears. 'Dad's asleep.'

'Excellent. He worked himself into a frenzy.'

'Yes, well you know what he's like. Not cheap though, is it?'

'No. Not one bit of this bloody trip is cheap. It's all outrageously expensive. Except for the Scooby Doo wagon, which is saving us thousands compared to a private jet.'

'True. Talking of which, better book it, now the dates are fixed.'

'Yes, do that. I'll book the hotel and spend the rest of the day figuring out how to convince your dad two grand, for two meetings, is a bargain.'

'Good luck with that, Mama lumps.'

...

'Momentous day today, chaps,' says Bruce, setting two cans of Special Brew on the coffee table, as he plonks himself onto what is now considered his preferred championship-viewing sofa.

'Told you England would win,' says Nigel, from the control centre at the back of the room. 'Leave my winnings on the table.'

'The championship, yes,' agrees Graham. 'But there's the small matter of the Grand Slam.'

'In the bag,' reckons Danny.

'Not so sure,' muses Tom. 'Ireland are a strong team.'

'Who's playing first?' says Daz.

'Scotland versus Italy.'

'Come on you Scots.'

'Should be a tense game, this.'

'Beers needed lads, before the drop kick?'

Half an hour into the match, Paula and I wander into the lounge bearing the first round of finger food. As predicted, Paula has elevated the menu these past six weeks from grub to gourmet, and today's platters are adorned with classic tomato and basil bruschetta, parmesan toasts and a garlicky mushroom creation, rendering my tuna sarnies and pork pies unquestionably 1980s.

'Good hands!'

'My God, that's a thunderous tackle.'

'It's the blood bin for him.'

'Wiping the floor with them, we are.'

'Friendly game,' I say, placing food on the coffee table.

'Rambunctious, is what it is,' says Bruce.

'Indeed. As the esteemed Churchill once said,' quotes Graham: '"Rugby is a game for hooligans played by gentlemen."'

'Lovely.'

'Another beer anybody?' offers Paula.

I gather samples of food for Nigel. 'You OK?' I whisper, leaning close to his ear.

'Fine,' he says, grinning.

As the France v Wales game kicks off, Paula and I refresh the table with home-made quiche, lemon sole goujons and spicy king prawns along with a gallon or two of booze. Checking on Nigel, I detect his catheter bag is full.

'Shall we empty that in the bathroom?'

'No, do it here,' he says, enthralled in the game.

'Sure?'

'Yes.'

I empty the urine from the bag into the jug kept solely for this task, as discreetly as possible. These boisterous blokes are distracted by the game and are unaware of what's happening, until Nigel draws attention to it.

'Don't mind Julie,' he says. 'She's just taking the piss.'

Groan. These jokes get better and better. Any response from a polite listener is smothered by the hollering associated with a successful conversion. Having attended one solitary rugby match in my life, understanding what a conversion is, represents the extent of my knowledge.

'Top man!'

'Teamwork makes the dream work.'

'Close fight, this, chaps.'

'Come on, Wales. Keep up.'

Wales, however, fail to keep up and the 20-18 victory for France is declared, as we caterers gather the leftover scraps of food, to make way for dessert. The climax of the championship, England v Ireland, is to be celebrated with a selection of bite-sized chunks of carrot, lemon drizzle and chocolate cake. As far as Paula is concerned, baking just the one cake is stupid. A minimum of three is standard.

'Ladies, you are spoiling us,' says Graham, as the delicacies hit the table.

'I'll say,' says Bruce, helping himself to a lump of all three cakes. 'Bring on the Lions tour in June.' He raises his can of beer in salute to Nigel. 'I'll warrant we'll receive an invitation, young man?'

All eyes flip to Nigel. Tom stops mid bite. Danny lifts the beer to his lips and halts it there and Daz freezes in his seat. There's a heartbeat of a pause. That established poker player's face betrays nothing. Will Nigel share his plans with Graham and Bruce?

'I won't be here, mate.'

There's the answer.

'Where're you bound, sir?' says Bruce.

Nigel inclines his chair and, with his habitual frankness, says, 'I'll be dead.'

A jumble of emotions flicker across their faces. Did I hear him right? Is he joking? Did he say what I thought he said? What does he mean? Dead?

'I'm off to Dignitas,' Nigel explains.

'Oh my,' exhales Graham.

'Mate?' chokes Bruce.

This conversation should take place without an audience. It's not fair for Graham and Bruce to be in the spotlight while they grapple with their feelings.

Gesturing to Paula, we gather the empty plates and flee.

'I'll fetch more drinks,' says Danny, grasping the point.

'I'll help,' says Daz, jumping to his feet.

Tom stays behind. There's no obvious excuse for him to leave.

'Awkward,' says Paula, from the safety of the kitchen.

'Poor buggers,' I say. 'Did you see their faces?'

'Better he tells them himself,' says Danny. 'They're old mates.'

'Give them a few minutes,' suggests Daz.

Like the carers, who are now aware of Nigel's plans, Bruce and Graham may struggle to understand why he would do this, now, when he conveys such an upbeat impression and seems more contented than he's been in months. He's coping so well. Never stopped joking. Never stopped laughing. What's changed?

There are no passionate cries of support for the teams in the final game of the championship. No praise for a slick ankle-tap tackle, or a strategically played box kick. No howls of 'Offside', or 'Where's the bloody Ref', clamouring from the lounge as England limps to defeat.

It is a pair of dismayed friends who shake Nigel by the hand at the end of the afternoon.

'A pleasure knowing you,' says Graham.

'An honour, sir,' says Bruce.

Bruce's normally ramrod-stiff shoulders sag like soggy washing as I escort them out. They falter at the door, perhaps unwilling to take that final step, knowing they'll never cross this threshold, never see Nigel, again. Graham places a hand on my arm. 'Take care of him. And yourself,' he whispers.

'Don't forget my winnings, lads,' cries Nigel from the lounge.

Graham swipes a hand across his eyes and emits a sorrowful moan. 'Remarkable man. Incorrigible. I will miss him.'

Bruce, unable to speak, clenches his fist and punches the air.

'I'll be in touch,' I say, closing the door.

...

Death hasn't shown its ugly face for a while. It has no need to. I can smell it. Suspended in the air, a lingering, all pervading stench. It has stolen the blush from Nigel's cheeks and shrouds his sleep in a profound stillness. There are moments I swear he's already lost. Each day he steps away from life and draws ever closer to death. No longer the repulsive phantom, spewing its scorn, this presence bears the promise of peace. This Death is his friend, his liberator.

Olivia from the hospice makes her final call. 'I am genuinely astonished by the change in you,' she says. 'I've never known you this calm.'

'Yes, I'm fine. No need for Lorazepam.'

'So, Julie tells me. You appear to be in control.'

'I am.'

'But you still have MND,' she says. 'And you are significantly weaker now, than just last month.'

She leans close to him. And as always, when she visits, Nigel relaxes. A serenity encompasses Olivia which I suspect results from her working with terminally ill patients. Or it may simply be her character. Her presence is soothing, and she creates a safe ambience. As soft and sweet as a marshmallow, there's nothing pointy or harsh about her. A baggy, cashmere jumper and ankle-length velvet skirt, enhance her curvy frame. Honey brown waves tumble erratically around a baby-smooth face. Her speech is melodious and unhurried. She lays a fleshy hand on Nigel's arm. 'Do you still intend to travel to Dignitas, Nigel?'

'I do.'

Olivia clasps her hands, as if in prayer. Soulful, chocolatey eyes pore into mine.

'I'm not sure he'll make the journey. I don't consider him well enough.'

'I'm worried too.'

'I'm not worried,' says Nigel. 'I'll be fine.'

'You're nothing if not determined, I'll give you that,' she says, taking hold of his hand. 'But, you know, there is another way.'

She has our attention.

'What's that?'

'Your condition has deteriorated significantly. Should you get an infection, we're not obliged to treat it. We don't need to prolong your life. We can ensure you are free of pain. And I suspect, if left alone, an infection would kill you.'

Nigel studies her face. Then mine. I hold my breath. He closes his eyes and sinks into the pillow. Could he change his mind? Is he considering it? Opening his eyes, he says, 'Got one in your bag?'

'What?'

'An infection.'

She inclines her head and raises her eyebrows. 'No.'

'Then I'm going to Dignitas.'

'I should've guessed,' she says.

Olivia accepts Nigel's decision and offers to provide us with a report to take with us to Switzerland, should anything happen to Nigel along the way, which may require medical intervention. It will summarise his condition and his wishes as outlined in the advanced directive to not prolong life.

Nigel thanks her for the care over the last ten years.

'You've been marvellous,' he says.

Olivia grasps his hand in both of hers. 'Nigel, it's been a privilege to care for you. You've had a huge impact on all of us. You always raise a laugh. You are, truly, an inspiration.'

'Thank you,' he mutters.

Swallowing the lump in my throat, I accompany Olivia to the door.

She lingers at the door and says, 'Julie, I am in awe of your strength and dedication in ensuring Nigel's had the best possible care.'

Stop. Don't be kind. I'll cry.

'Best of luck,' she says. 'And please, do consider counselling when this is over. Call me any time.'

I manage a humble 'Thank you' and close the door on the doctor for the final time.

'Come on buggerlugs, out of bed.'

I wrap the sling around him and hoist him from the bed. 'You left Olivia in no doubt.'

'Yes,' he says, dangling.

'A natural death would be better though, wouldn't it?'

'True, but who knows when a nice little infection will come along and kill me? Won't risk the wait. I want to die happy and smiling, while I still can. Not when this disease decides my time is up.'

'OK.'

'And anyway. 'I'm excited about our city break.'

'You blow my mind, Nig. I always knew you were amazing, but you beat all records.'

I manoeuvre the hoist to lower him into his chair. 'Thank you,' he says.

'You're welcome. Not going to leave you hanging there, am I?'

'No, I mean, thank you for being my wife all these years. You're wonderful. You've made me very happy.'

This expression of tenderness takes me by surprise and a surge of love locks in my throat. I find distraction in releasing the sling from the hoist and fight the swell of tears which blind me.

'And thanks for looking after me. None of this was supposed to happen. Not part of our plan. I'm sorry.'

Sorry. As if he could prevent any of this.

'Oh, Nig.' I cradle him close to my chest and kiss his head. Jean Paul Gaultier today's choice of aftershave. Lovely. He wraps his arms around my waist, and we hold each other as we yearn for all we have lost.

'Are you determined to go through with this Nig?' I ask. I know the answer. It's been the same every day since I first asked in September. I need to hear it, daily.

'Definitely.'

'OK.'

He pulls away from me and eyes full of love seek mine. 'You are with me on this?'

'Yes. I am. But I'm going to lose you.' I sit on his knee and cradle him as I rest my head on his shoulder. 'I'm not ready to live without you.'

He strokes my hair. 'It's the best thing for me.'

I kiss his neck. 'I love you.'

Immersed in our embrace, my warm breath on his neck, his arm at my waist, one hand cupping my face. 'I know you do. You're the only one who could talk me out of it.'

I take a second to absorb his words. I wasn't expecting him to say that. What to do with this knowledge? Persuade him to change his mind? Beg him to stay with us a bit longer, in the hope of a natural death? Would it be fair to ask him? I consider how he has dealt with MND. Not one complaint in ten long years. Not one moment's self-pity. He has scoffed at this vile disease and fought every battle with unparalleled courage. Then, with the certain knowledge MND will crush his spirit as mercilessly as it has violated his body, he calls a halt. He denies it victory. He takes control. I reflect on the change in him. The joy he has known since October, the enhanced quality of life because he is in control of how and when it ends.

How he must love me to trust me with this responsibility. To risk me changing his mind. And if I did, would it be for him or me? Am I willing to condemn him to endure the torture of a living death? Could I allow him to shrivel as his soul is snatched from him? Could I stand by while the man I adore is plagued by eternal suffering?

The noblest sacrifice any of us could ever face, is to give one's life for another. Nigel is prepared to go one step further. To sacrifice his death.

'Will you try to talk me out of it?' he says.

As I sink into those luminous sea-green pools, the quivering beat of my heart declares me the luckiest woman in the world.

'No, my darling, I won't talk you out of it. I love you too much.'

30
TWENTY-FIVE DAYS LEFT TO LIVE

Golden rays of spring sunshine seep into Nigel's room and wake him with a tender kiss. Outside, new growth flourishes, and delicate buds open to the radiant warmth, as if embracing hope and the promise of summer. A summer Nigel will not see.

'Morning, darling. A bit of sunbathing on the patio for you today, I reckon. You need some colour in those cheeks.'

'Morning,' says Nigel, squinting against the light. He inclines the bed and fires up his iPad. '1 April.'

'Don't I know it.' April. Already. I curl his fingers around the first cuppa of the day. 'Any practical jokes planned?'

'No, but,' he giggles as a thought occurs to him. 'I wish I'd asked Ellie to make me an advent calendar.'

'It's April Fool not Christmas.'

His imagination shifts gear, and he snorts, spluttering tea down his chin. I grab the cup before he dissolves into meltdown, lean him forward and dab his face. 'What do you mean?'

'Well,' he warbles once the chortling subsides. 'I could open a new door as I count down to D Day.'

Reluctant to ask but I force myself. 'D Day?'

'Yeah,' he says, eyes sparkling with mischief. 'Dying day.'

'Bloody hell, Nig.'

'It'd be brilliant,' he gurgles. 'A picture of the Grim Reaper behind one door, a bottle of poison behind another. Skull and crossbones in another. A graveyard should be in there somewhere. What else?'

'Pair of feet on a slab? Label hanging from a big toe?' I suggest.

'Yes, clever. How about, on the 25th, a coffin with the sign David Nigel Casson. RIP.'

'My God, what are you like?' I chuckle, despite myself. 'Nobody but you would think of that.'

'You've got to laugh, eh?' he says, as I hand him back his tea.

'I suppose so. It's like you can't wait for it to happen, Nig.'

'I can't,' he says, without hesitation. 'It's time to go.'

He grows weaker each day. Any longer and he'll have no choice but to remain alive. Journeying to Switzerland would be impossible. And yet, as his physical strength deserts him, his inner strength intensifies. Focused on the challenge he faces, he is committed to embracing death, cheerfully and on his own terms.

He scrutinises me as I line up the medication for the trip. Lorazepam? No Lorazepam? Stupid question. Bung them in the bag with their 'pam' mates. Won't leave those phenomenal blue lifesavers behind.

'I won't need them,' says Nigel.

'You might. You never know.'

'I do know,' he insists.

'They're not heavy. I'm packing them.'

'I'm telling you; I won't need them.'

Some may call it forthright, others bullying. I don't care. 'Fine. I might bloody need them. They're coming.'

'I give in.'

'As you should. Now, come on. Let's park you outside in this glorious sunshine.'

···

All the plans for Nigel's final day are concluded and we are immersed in preparations for his memorial do. Oh, I do love a 'do.' Normally. A wedding or a birthday bash. Any kind of party to be honest: dinner, garden, pool, hello or goodbye, new pad, old pad, met a new fella, dumped a fella, passed or failed exams, no reason whatsoever party. You name it. Shove a virgin notebook and a quality ballpoint in my hand and I will create lists of what to do when, who's to do what, and how to do the whole lot in between. Orderliness will emerge from disorder and pandemonium will be parcelled into a framework of prioritised boxes. Usually.

Planning my husband's memorial while he is still alive is new to me. Rather than play the lead protagonist I settle into the role of collaborator and allow Nigel to be chief planner. The kids and others become co-conspirators and we sculpt a spectacular day. Our first family conference combines Ellie's evening shift with a chance to grab a takeaway of pepperoni and Bolognese pizzas, doner kebabs, chips and the mandatory garlic bread with extra garlic for his Lordship.

'I can't have a miserable do, with everybody wearing black,' he says.

'What then?'

'Tell them to wear yellow,' he says.

'Yellow?' echoes Craig.

I gulp down a lump of pizza before it chokes me. 'There's not a woman in the world who would choose to wear yellow.'

'I know,' he grins, a wicked glint in his eye.

'You're such a bastard, Dad,' says Becky.

'Yeah, I know that, too.'

'You've got to be kidding,' says Ellie. 'We'll look like a bunch of bloody bananas.'

'Or a flock of Big Bird muppets,' says Craig.

'Could we wear a touch of yellow?' I ask, desperate for a compromise. 'Like a yellow scarf, handbag, shoes. That kind of thing.'

'Yeah, I could wear a black T-shirt with a big yellow smiley face on the front,' suggests Craig.

'That'd be awesome,' agrees Becky.

'I could live with yellow accessories,' says Ellie.

We're wearing him down. We're winning. 'OK,' he says. 'Tell everybody to wear what they like, but there must be a bit of yellow. A ray of sunshine.'

Relieved, I fetch Nigel another beer and we greedily tuck into the food before tackling the next item on the agenda: music. Not my forte. This, apart from the single request of, 'Anything except Frank Sinatra and *My Way*' I leave to them.

'Pink Floyd's a must, Dad,' says Craig, shoving a slab of Bolognese pizza in his mouth. 'We were brought up on them.'

We wait for him to finish the job of chewing the last bit of doner kebab. Foolish choice, a messy challenge at the best of times. 'Yes,' he says. 'Brilliant idea. Carry me in to *Comfortably Numb*.'

'So long as the funeral directors deliver you home in time,' I point out. 'Otherwise, it'll be an urn full of sand from the beach and the odd crab's claw.'

'Ha. Funny.'

Ellie reaches for the wine. 'Isn't that song about drugs?'

'Does it matter?' says Becky. 'Top me up while you're at it, Ellie.'

Nigel bites on a chip. 'Don't think so. Anyway, it doesn't matter. The lyrics still work.'

'What should we play while your visual tribute is rolling?' I ask.

'That's easy,' he says. 'Bob Dylan's *Forever Young*.'

'Ah, the getting arrested song,' says Ellie, referring to the time when Nigel was apprehended by the police, as he slumped in the car, snoring his head off, engine running, Bob Dylan belting out *Forever Young* at full volume.

'How many songs should there be?' Becky asks, attacking the last piece of pepperoni.

'Some chips here if anybody fancies them,' says Ellie, waving a polystyrene carton in the air.

'One more during the service and another as we all file out,' I say.

'Pink Floyd's *Goodbye Cruel World* next,' decrees Nigel.

'Yes,' says Becky. 'In case people aren't wrecked by this point. That should sort them out.'

'What to end with?' asks Nigel. 'Something lively.'

Craig bursts into song, 'Don't worry, be happy.'

'Nah.'

'I know. The one you always played when you came home pissed on Saturday afternoons,' says Craig. '*A Fistful of Dollars*.'

'Perfect.'

I check my notes. We're doing well.

'Who's doing the introduction and stuff?' says Craig. 'You?'

'No,' I say. 'I considered it but changed my mind. I'll be doing a personal tribute though. The celebrant who officiated at Grandad Ron's funeral is doing it.'

'George? Yes, I cleaned his windows when he lived up Newby way.'

'Well, he's coming to discuss it next week. Join us if you can.'

Becky plonks her glass of wine on the table. 'He knows you're off to Dignitas?'

'Yes,' says Nigel, beaming.

'Bloody hell,' says Craig, flopping against the back of the settee. 'Do you trust him?'

'We've no choice.'

'He can't plan many services with people before they set off for Dignitas,' says Ellie.

'None, I suspect.'

'How will that conversation pan out, I wonder?' says Becky.

Nigel can do nothing to quash the budding burble in his throat. 'I'm planning on telling him –'

'Uh oh, here we go,' says Craig, as the burbling becomes a torrent.

Ellie leaps to her feet and assumes the 'ready for anything' position beside his chair.

'To tell him the –' A whinny now.

'Won't be long,' says Becky.

Craig points an accusing finger at Becky. 'See what you started Becky.'

'Ram it, Craig.'

The exchange exacerbates the hilarity.

'Nig,' I say. 'Calm down.'

Ellie steadies him as he inhales lungsful of air and, finally, he stammers, 'The baby polar bear joke.'

That's it, we reach full trumpeting level.

'Wish I could be here for that,' says Becky. 'Best of luck you lot.'

I clear the debris from the table while Nigel composes himself. I could clean the house, do the ironing and decorate a room or two before he's recovered. 'Anybody like another drink? Wine, girls? Craig?' I won't ask Nigel, he's not up to speaking yet.

Ellie and Becky raise their glasses.

'Not for me,' says Craig. 'Are we nearly done? Dad's knackered.'

'Not surprised,' says Becky.

Nigel manages a weary 'I'm OK.'

'Won't be long,' I say. 'Who intends to speak at the service, apart from me?'

'Me,' says Becky, without hesitation.

Nigel inclines his chair. 'Are you piping up Becky?'

'*Pipe up*?' I hoot. 'I haven't heard that expression for years.'

She glowers at him. 'Of course, I'm piping up. I've already planned what to say.'

'And me,' says Ellie. 'I intend to pipe up as well. But I've no idea yet what to say.'

Nigel chuckles and his shoulders quake. This could be dangerous. I call a halt and demand we all pipe down.

Nigel ignores me. 'What about you Craig? Are you piping up?'

He shudders at the prospect. 'Not a bloody chance. I couldn't speak in front of people. I'll write something for George to read.'

'Gonna be a fab do,' says Nigel. 'Shame I'll miss it.'

...

As Scarborough's sole four-star hotel, the lounge at the Crown Spa wears its unchanged lacklustre décor with confidence. We order coffee and head for a corner grouping near the bar and sink into the aged-leather mulberry tub chairs.

'Two weddings and a funeral, we've hosted here,' I say, surveying the familiar surroundings.

'Isn't that a film?' says Paula.

'It is. Although you're probably thinking of *Four Weddings and a Funeral*.'

'Yes I am.'

'Different film.'

Behind us, the gurgling coffee machine sputters boiling water into our waiting cafetiere as the barista batters spent grounds into the knock box.

Paula winces. 'Is that level of violence necessary, do you reckon?'

'Wouldn't want to get on the wrong side of him.'

'Hope it's worth the abuse.'

Our coffee arrives as Louise, the Events Manager, joins us.

'Mrs Casson?'

'Julie, hi.'

'And?'

'Hi, Paula.'

'Sisters?'

'Yes.'

'Lovely. I'm Louise.'

Late thirties, with a wild pumpkin mop framing a freckly, kittenish face, Louise smiles as she sits opposite. She tucks clumpy curls behind wing nut ears and taps her iPad into life with a tablet pen. Despite those ears doing an excellent job of taming her hair, I'd have had them pinned.

The barista pummels more grounds into their grave.

'Jesus,' hisses Paula, glaring behind her with murderous intent.

'Now,' Louise says, 'let me find your email. Ah, here we are. So, Consort Suite and Imperial Suite, 20th May. Correct?'

I mentally cross my fingers. Nigel's ashes should be back by then. 'Yes, that's right. We'd like the Imperial Suite from 12.30 pm., followed by the ceremony in the Consort Suite at 2.00 pm.'

'Excellent. What's the nature of the occasion?'

'It's a memorial. If you set the room up as you would a wedding. Tables at the front. A lectern for speakers. Central aisle and as many rows of chairs as possible for guests.'

'The room comfortably holds 120 people.'

'There'll be at least 150.'

'I'd guess more,' adds Paula.

'We'll confirm numbers nearer the time. People will stand, if necessary,' I say.

'And the name?' says Louise.

'Sorry?'

'Of the person whose memorial it is. So, the notices are prepared, and so on.'

Oh shit. What should I say? I can hardly announce that it's my husband's memorial, but he's not dead yet. I dive in with, 'Again, could I confirm nearer the time? If we could sort the arrangements today and perhaps consider the menu options?'

A perplexed frown creases Louisa's forehead and those ears flush pink.

'Should we choose the food now or take the menus away and confirm later?' asks Paula, assisting in the bombardment.

Behind the bar, yet more grounds are assaulted.

'For God's sake!' spits Paula.

'Oh, and it will be a free bar,' I say, in the hope this snippet of information will deflect her attention from the memorial recipient.

'Also,' interjects Paula, 'if the guests adjourn to the bar following the ceremony, how long would you need to set up tables for the buffet in the Consort Suite?'

'Could we discuss your audio system and visual display facilities? I'm hoping to run a continuous loop of photographs, as a tribute, throughout the day. My son-in-law is our technical guru. Perhaps he could discuss things with your technician?'

Louise responds to our questions and records our requirements on her iPad. I suspect she is irritated by the sections in her pro-forma which, for now, must read 'to be confirmed'. She hides it well and asks us to contact her within the week with our food and other outstanding options. She won't be anywhere near as irritated as Paula, however, who, I fear, may leap over the bar and slay the barista with her bare hands unless we escape right now.

'You need to make sure he's not working on 20 May,' she says as we race to the door.

'Don't worry. Nobody will be drinking coffee at Nig's do.'

...

The waking hours of his remaining days are spent composing two messages. First, his final post to his 425 friends on Facebook.

'What are you planning to say?'

'I've got some ideas. I want to leave them laughing.'

'Not like you,' I joke.

He drafts and redrafts his message, adds a word here, deletes a word there, until 'Here,' he says, 'what do you think?'

'Wow, Nig. That's powerful. Quite the farewell.'

'You think?'

'Definitely. Don't know about leaving them laughing. You'll make them weep.'

'Oh,' he says, his brow creased with consternation. 'Should I change it?'

I kiss his head. 'Not a single word. It's perfect.'

'OK,' he smiles. 'It's here on my iPad. Post it when I'm dead.'

'You don't want to post it before you die?'

'No,' he says. 'I won't spend my last few hours glued to Facebook. I'd prefer to be with you and the kids.'

'Well, I think it will have a hell of an impact.'

His message to the guests at his memorial and the many tasks I must perform once he is no more, consume our afternoons. A spanking new notebook and pen are purchased for this specific purpose. Yes, it may be more time efficient to input straight into my laptop or phone, but this dinosaur prefers pen and paper.

Inform SKY, BT, broadband. Be sure to claim the insurance. Let DWP know. Update utility and bank accounts.

'Check the bank daily,' he says.

'Every day?'

'Yes.'

'Are you expecting a financial crisis like 2008?'

'You never know. Assume scams. Don't be caught out.'

Struggling to perceive such diligent behaviour, I nevertheless promise to check the bank every single day.

He dictates snippets of what the celebrant will read at his memorial as the thoughts occur to him. I draft the composition with care, conscious of Nigel's determination to leave an optimistic, no regrets message. A message bursting with characteristic wisecracks and the cast-iron certainty of raising a smile on the faces of those privileged to know him.

He opens with, 'Have I told you the one about the baby polar bear?' There will be few unfamiliar with the joke, and none by the end of the day. He hopes we're wearing a touch of yellow and jokes how he's speaking from the box on the table.

He confirms his determination to 'take back control of what's left of my life.' To 'die a happy man, still smiling, on my terms.' He assures us he is at one with his actions. Pleased to have found the cure. He describes an active, fun-filled, stimulating and, except for the loss of his first wife, a wonderful and happy life. Proud to be part of a loving family, with siblings who remain as close now as when they were children and lucky enough to share a long and happy marriage with me, his wife and best friend.

Our three children and four grandchildren receive a special message: 'Be happy. Don't be sad. Get on with your lives. Make the most of it. Have loads of fun, never waste a moment, look after each other, guard your money and don't be fooled into believing life owes you any favours. Life isn't fair. There's always a kick in the bollocks around the corner. But that doesn't stop life from being wonderful.'

Apart from playing off scratch, he says he has achieved everything he set out to achieve. 'To you golfers,' he says, 'I hope all of you will one day win the Casson Shield. If your ball lands in Casson's Copse, it's mine.'

Finally, he thanks us all for the laughs and for sharing his life. We are urged to raise our glasses and to give pots of money to the MND Association, the box on the memory table, right next to his urn. He ends with the sentiment he chose to live by and instructs us all to: 'Keep smiling.'

When Nigel is satisfied with his messages, the venue, music and order of service, he closes his eyes and relaxes against his pillow.

'I'm ready. Bring it on.'

31
THE GOODBYES

'He's five minutes away,' says Ellie, placing her phone on the table.

'Take me outside,' says Nigel, 'I want to see it.'

'Me too,' I say. 'Come on.'

Five minutes gives us time to bundle Nigel outside to await the arrival of the motorhome which will take us to Zurich. Daz, our designated driver, kindly offered to collect it from the owner and drive it to Scarborough in readiness for our departure.

'Our very own *Scooby Doo* wagon is here,' I say, noting the lumbering progress of the motorhome as it rattles to a halt. 'Seems a bit cumbersome.'

'How'd it go?' demands Ellie before Daz's feet hit the ground.

'Hello to you too,' he says. 'How'd what go?'

Daz grabs his bag from the seat and swings it onto his back. Had he a wild mop of hair, he could double for Shaggy from *Scooby Doo*. Casually dressed in loose T-shirt and comfortable old combat shorts, he's the embodiment of nonchalant. He signals hello to Nigel. 'Fancy a peek inside?'

'Please.'

He opens the passenger door to the motorhome and operates the mechanism to release the ramp.

'When you picked it up from the owner,' Ellie urges, 'did she ask where we were going?'

'Yes.'

'You didn't say Switzerland, did you?' says Ellie. 'Tell me you stuck to the script. You didn't blab we're going to Zurich?'

'He's not daft, Ellie,' I intervene.

Daz stops what he's doing and faces Ellie, hands on hips. 'Yes, course I did, Elea-*nor*. I informed her we're headed for Dignitas with your dying dad and perhaps she'd like to ring the police.'

Nigel giggles. 'Like it.'

Ellie glares at him. 'What did you say, exactly?'

'That we are touring France, and we'll maybe slip into Germany.'

'Why Germany?' I ask.

'She needed an idea of mileage, and Germany is next door to Switzerland. Thus, our proximity is explained.'

'Oh, OK. Cool,' says Ellie relaxing. 'Sorry.'

'No probs, *Nor*,' he says, nudging her with his elbow.

'He's as accomplished a liar as you, Ellie.' I say, clambering into the motorhome. 'Come on Nig, into the Scooby Doo wagon you go.'

It's not exactly the iconic, supercool, mystery machine of *Scooby Doo* lore, promising excitement and adventure. Nor does it sport aqua blue and green chassis, embellished with bright orange flowers. It's an imposing, practical, unadorned piece of kit. There's an access ramp, ample seats and a safe place to anchor Nigel's chair. Two sleeping areas, one offering profiling bed with ceiling hoist and track leading to a shower and toilet. I survey the adapted space within the cab. Hardly the luxurious private jet of which we dreamed. Still, it will suffice. My thoughts veer to the owner's disabled son. This transport gives him the freedom to travel, to enjoy holidays with family and to be like everybody else. For us, this vehicle will carry Nigel to his death.

'It's perfect, isn't it?' he says, with a smile as bright as dawn on a dazzling summer's day.

'Couldn't be better, Nig,' I lie. 'We couldn't wish for more.'

'What shall we call it?' says Nigel. 'It needs a name.'

'Great idea,' says Daz.

'Scooby?' I suggest.

'No. Mabel,' says Nigel. 'She looks like a Mabel.'

'Love it,' says Daz.

'We'll start packing Mabel tomorrow, Mum,' says Ellie.

I agree. 'Yes. We must. There's scarcely any time left.'

Time only for goodbyes.

•••

If a secret is that which you tell one person at a time, then somebody has been busy. As the date of our departure draws near, the stream of people intensifies. Most are edgy and uncertain of how to behave in this unique and challenging situation. Like the granting of an audience with royalty, they're honoured and terrified at the same time.

'I don't know what to say,' they declare.

'Don't worry, he'll make it easy for you,' I tell them.

Gamby, his long-suffering golfing friend, forever the butt of Nigel's teasing, is tasked with ensuring fellow golfers attend his memorial. I know Nigel will tease him with one last gag, yet their final handshake will convey a sincere friendship more powerfully than words.

Glyn fidgets with his keys and taps repeatedly on the island worktop, dancing from one foot to another like a boxer limbering up before a round. 'Shit. I'm not sure I can do this,' he says.

Having directed so many down that corridor I assure him he'll be fine. Tinkling laughter, not plaintive wailing, is what resonates from Nigel's room. He talks of inconsequential, normal things, perhaps recalls some shared activity and behaves as if he'll be meeting you again next week. When it's time for that final kiss, that closing handshake, that ultimate farewell, he somehow drags a witty remark from his humour stable. 'Have you time to tattoo "may contain nuts" on my scrotum?' he says to tattooist Dan's departing back.

'He makes it so easy,' say his nephews, smiling in admiration and, like others before them, leave with the enduring memory of Nigel's inimitable, gleeful giggling.

True, there are those who struggle to keep a grip on their composure. Some, like Glyn, need a hug. Some hold it together until they've fled the house, others, especially the carers, weep inconsolably. Those unable to express their thoughts follow up their visit with an email or card, where they find the means to tell Nigel, eloquently and with sincere emotion, the impact he has had on their lives.

The final days are devoted to family. Craig, Charlotte and the girls spend the evening with us, then Danny, Ellie and their boys. Becky comes home on leave. Tracey flies in from Tenerife and joins us, along with Mel and Derek, Les, Sally, Paula and Tom for a takeaway and a few drinks. When Nigel retires to bed, those who are not travelling to Switzerland spend a few precious minutes alone with him. Each finds his or her way to say that last, agonising goodbye. Whatever Nigel says in response, be it a spot of advice, an enlightening snippet of wisdom, a request, a thank you or a characteristic wisecrack, remains locked in their hearts.

On the morning of 22 April 2017, the family gather in the lounge. They are subdued as they wait, like guests in a receiving line, to share a few more seconds with Nigel.

Grief is carved into the bones of Tracey and Melanie's faces as they embrace their brother for the final time. Pressing fists to their mouths to staunch their sobs, they fail to stifle the silent tears while they witness their brother Les and the procession of mourners bid Nigel farewell. Derek cradles the weeping sisters in his protective arms. Paula, on the edge of crumbling, is supported through the ordeal, by Tom. Danny guides his sons. Brave young Tom grips Nigel's hand and attempts a smile as he mutters, 'Bye Grandad.' Ben, anxious in social settings and traumatised by Grandad's plans, hangs back. Nigel reaches for his hand, draws him near and hugs him close. He whispers something in Ben's ear. His words are smothered by the sniffling in the room.

It's time.

Before making to leave, Nigel halts and asks for the other, adored, member of the family. 'Where's Bodger?'

Becky carries Bodger from the kitchen and nestles him on Nigel's knee where he peers, in his doggy way, into Nigel's eyes, perhaps sensing the magnitude of this moment. Under normal circumstances he would scramble to the ground, but if any dog can tune into a pervading atmosphere, it's a miniature schnauzer, and Bodger stays put. He licks Nigel's trembling hand as he moves to stroke his head.

'Bye, little fella,' he murmurs.

A heartfelt moan of, 'Oh God,' emanates from somewhere in the room.

'Look after him, won't you?'

'Always,' I gulp.

Now, it's time.

'Thanks, you lot, for being my family,' he says. 'I've had a hell of a ride. Now it's time to get off.' With a final swagger, he performs a 360-degree swivel. 'Take care of each other,' he yells, zooming down the corridor to the ramp.

The family rush outside and crowd onto the pavement to find a spot to wave us off.

While Nigel is helped into the motorhome, Craig grabs a battered pillow from his van.

'What the hell is that for?' I say, gawping at the offensive object, yellowed with age and sweat.

'My neck. I'm not comfy without it.'

'Don't imagine you're taking that into the hotel. Not a chance.'

Wheelchair anchored securely. Becky in the front alongside Daz. Craig, Ellie and me, strapped into seats I'm convinced will provide not a smidgen of comfort within the hour, never mind twenty. Nigel bubbles with excitement and waves like he's setting off on the holiday of a lifetime. In a way, I suppose he is.

The cluster outside waves back, cheerful expressions forced onto faces still swollen from sobbing. Derek presses the palm of his hand against the window. Danny holds Bodger with one hand and salutes Nigel with the other. Tom respectfully taps the side of the vehicle. Paula, Mel, Tracey and Sally, wave, blow kisses and wipe away torrents of tears.

Les stands apart from the rest, hands in pockets. His eyes meet Nigel's. Their gaze locks. After the briefest pause, the two brothers exchange a virtually imperceptible nod. That simple nod encapsulates their entire lives. During their lifetimes they have shared good times and bad. Worked, played, got mind-numbingly drunk and laughed and cried. The years have formed a brotherly bond, so intense, it can be expressed in a single nod. It is one of the most moving gestures I have ever witnessed.

'Come on Daz. Let's do it,' says Nigel.

Daz cranks the engine. The beast clatters awake. Pots, pans and cutlery rattle in cupboards as we shudder into gear and lurch forward. We're off. I watch the waving gathering as we rumble up the street. They'll spend the rest of today devouring the food Paula has organised and demolishing the barrel-loads of wine in the garage. All except Ben, who is already striding away from the scene, alone.

Never having travelled in a motorhome, I'm surprised how the vehicle sways like a boat in a choppy sea. I had visualised ambling around, making a sandwich, pouring a glass of wine. Not a bit of it. In your seat – seatbelt on – is the only way to travel safely inside one of these. I tighten my seatbelt and attempt to find a comfortable spot.

Craig shuffles in his seat. 'You do know,' he says, 'if this thing crashes, Dad will be the sole survivor.'

'Typical,' I say.

'That would piss you right off, wouldn't it, Dad?'

'Certainly would.'

'We won't crash,' insists Daz from the driving seat. 'Have confidence.'

'Yeah,' says Becky. 'Shut up you lot. Daz is on it.'

'What happens when Ellie's driving?' says Craig.

'Shut yer face, cheeky bastard,' says Ellie. 'Or we'll make *you* drive.'

'Well then we would definitely crash,' admits Craig.

We each find a way to stomach the gruelling twenty-hour journey. Becky plays the part of Daz's wing-woman: chattering, supporting, keeping him focused. Ellie provides him with occasional short breaks and carries us onwards while he rests. Craig takes his revolting pillow to one of the sleeping compartments and spends fifty percent of the time dreaming in the land of nod. Nigel, without the aid of a solitary Lorazepam, slumbers peacefully most of the way. I close my eyes when their stinging becomes intolerable and listen to the incessant jangling within the cab, wobbling in time with the motion. As we hurtle ever closer to our destination and are swallowed by the shadows of the night, its consoling blackness does little to obscure the blinding and terrifying images of what is about to happen.

32

THE HOTEL AND THE DOCTOR

The imposing Dolder Grand Hotel, suspended 200 metres above Zurich's vibrant city centre, is not your average 'Premier Inn' type of establishment. Apart from treating its guests to breathtaking views of the city, the Alps and lake, it boasts 175 beyond-luxurious rooms and suites, suitable for royalty, wealthy celebs and uber-rich nobodies. The stylish restaurants, dishing up innovative, gourmet cuisine worthy of two Michelin stars, are considered world class. Its Spa, a mere 4000 square metres, offers those who are not in the mood to thrash around the hotel's nine-hole golf course, or lob some balls on one of its five tennis courts, the opportunity to indulge in a host of calming wellness and meditative diversions, or any degree of punishing fitness workout you could concoct. Should you consider all this a tad dull, you could always stroll through the opulent and matchless interior and marvel at any one of the hundred-plus works of art dotted around the walls, with the odd original from Takashi Murakami and Salvador Dali chucked into the pot.

The Dolder Grand is not the kind of place where you rock up in a battered old motorhome.

In the afternoon of 23 April 2017, our grungy, whacked-out carcass of a vehicle, as dishevelled and bleary-eyed as its passengers, lurches up the steep and winding hill towards the palatial splendour of this magical domain. Once at the top, Daz swings her lumbering bulk around, intent on reversing to the entrance.

'Bloody hell. The car park's full of Porsches and Bentleys. You're not driving Mabel in there,' cries Ellie.

'We look like druggies from *Breaking Bad's* RV,' says Craig, leaping from the vehicle. 'I'll guide you in Daz.'

Craig races into the car park and cracks on with his aircraft marshaller impersonation, while Daz rams the engine into reverse. Mabel screams in protest as she bulldozes her way to the lavish foyer of this elegant hotel with all the subtlety of a Challenger tank sneaking up on a sniper.

'Sounds like her belt's squeaking, Daz,' says Nigel.

Inside the vehicle, we girls feign invisibility by shielding our faces with our hands and peeping through our fingers at the affluent, designer-dripping punters scrutinising this unexpected scene, whilst sipping their Dom Perignon from Baccarat flutes upon the stylish terrace. We don't need to read lips, just horrified faces, to guess the dialogue.

'Gypsies, do you suppose? Wandered unwittingly away from their traditional laybys?' 'Lottery winners, perhaps?' 'Surely they've come to the wrong place?'

The hotel's 'one of a kind' concierge surges from the hotel lobby, flapping his arms as wildly as Craig, as Mabel grinds to a halt.

'We're guests,' Craig explains to the disbelieving, though polite, concierge. 'Booked in.'

'Better sort it, Julie,' suggests Nigel.

I leap from the vehicle and waft our reservation in the concierge's face. He makes a good job of masking his surprise and his training in dealing with all manner of patrons is obvious, although he directs us, with undisguised urgency, to park this abomination at the back. The rear car park is also bursting with Porsches, Bentleys, Mercs and one or two BMWs. Not a single motorhome. Imagine that.

Ellie and I help Nigel out, while Daz, Craig and Becky retrieve the bags. A bellman, pushing a gleaming brass, plushily carpeted, birdcage luggage trolley appears as his colleague departs with a similar contraption bearing a complete set of matching Gucci luggage. Our Debenham trolley bags and collection of Sainsbury's bags for life, Tesco wine and Morrisons carriers project a cheap and shabby image in comparison.

Becky and Craig check Mabel for anything we've missed, and Craig appears at the door with his pillow under his arm.

I glare at him. 'No.'

'But –'

'They have pillows at this hotel.'

His gaze travels to our supermarket branded luggage and I concede he has a point. Still. There are limits.

'No.'

I win. He throws the pillow back into the vehicle. I'll ask Daz to ditch it before he takes Mabel home.

Relief floods the concierge's features when I explain this eyesore will not litter the car park for more than an hour.

'Are you sure you won't stay a bit longer, Daz?' I ask.

'No. I'll grab a drink and set off.'

'Where will you sleep?' says Becky. 'Couldn't you stay at least until tonight? Rest your head a bit?'

'Stay overnight,' says Nigel. 'You've driven non-stop.'

'No, no,' he insists. 'I'll park up and sleep before I reach the tunnel.'

We weary travellers take our stinking bodies into the sumptuous reception and bar area and sink into cushioned seating so deliciously squashy it could compete with Craig's pillow. Light cascades through the wall of elaborate arched windows, bathing the lofty room with sunshine and warmth.

'You didn't say it was this posh,' says Craig.

'It was dark last time we were here,' says Becky.

'Eh?'

'Never mind,' she says. 'Anyway, we didn't come into this bit.'

'Have you never stayed in a five-star hotel, Craig?' says Ellie.

'No.'

'Might as well start with the best,' says Nigel.

'Any chance of a drink?' says Ellie.

I drag myself to my feet. 'I'll register first. I understand we're offered a complimentary drink while they make sure the rooms are ready. Won't be long.'

That must be a Warhol, I muse, studying the four faces of Marilyn Monroe hanging behind Reception. The only other works of his I'm familiar with, are 'Campbell's Soup', which I find ridiculous, and 'After the Party', a print of which hangs in my dining room. The receptionist logs my card details and explains someone will be along in half an hour to usher us to our rooms and show us how everything works. What can be so difficult? I wonder. When I return to the bar, a waiter is taking our drinks order and I add a gin and tonic to the list in the hope it will revive me.

We made it. My bedraggled, stinking, exhausted family are installed in the bar of Zurich's finest hotel. It's mindboggling. Here we are. We have travelled over 800 miles from Scarborough to Zurich, with a severely ill, disabled, yet contented, man. And, as it transpires, had fewer problems along the way than when Becky and I carried out the recce.

Our drinks arrive. I curl Nigel's fingers around his beer and slip a straw into the top. Nigel, the single member of our group not dropping from sleep deprivation, lifts the bottle of beer towards our family circle. 'Cheers,' he says.

'Cheers,' we cry, as one.

'Thanks for everything Daz,' says Nigel. 'You've been fantastic.'

'Couldn't have done it without you,' says Craig. 'I would never have got us here.'

Daz downs his pint of orange juice in seconds, stands and bats the compliments away. 'Don't be daft. It's nothing.'

'It is, mate,' insists Craig, shaking his hand.

'Safe journey home,' I say, embracing him. 'Be sure to stop and rest.'

'Thanks Daz,' says Ellie with a hug. 'Take care on the way home.'

'I'll walk you to the car park,' says Becky.

'Thank you, again,' says Nigel. 'Good luck.'

Daz shakes Nigel's hand. His jaw is clamped shut. Swallowing hard, he juts out his chin and flees from the bar.

This scene is familiar to us now: the 'never see him again' moment, the final goodbye. It occurs to me we may be developing some form of immunity, a protective shell shielding us from its enormity. Craig draws a long breath as Daz disappears, before exhaling with a guttural cough. Ellie buries her face in her gin. I chew at the thumb nail of one hand and rub at Nigel's leg, with the other. No, we're not immune.

When Becky returns a few minutes later, she hands her dad a piece of paper with the words Daz was unable to utter in person, written upon it. Nigel absorbs the contents and returns the note to Becky with a faint smile. She folds it in half and slots it in her bag. What's written there is nobody else's business.

When we are ushered to our rooms and the concierge explains how the fixtures and fittings are operated by the iPad on the desk, I am pleased Ellie and Becky are in the room adjoining ours. Lights, TV, blinds, heat. He demonstrates the magic with such gusto he must have shares in Apple. I hope the girls are listening as not a single instruction penetrates my skull and technophobe Craig has no chance. Oh, for the love of switches. There must be alternatives for us Luddites.

With our carers hats on, Ellie and I inspect the room's facilities. The mobile hoist, sling and disabled shower chair are present, as requested. The settee and two armchairs need removing as they're in the way. Six more pillows please. I'll never prop him up without. No grab rail in the toilet. The floor-to-ceiling frosted glass doors into the separate toilet and shower are heavy and awkward and could block the hoist.

'What if we hold the door out of the way and swing the hoist to swivel him into the toilet?' I ask.

'It's a tight squeeze,' says Ellie. 'It'll take two of us.'

The image of Patsy and Eddie, making a total arse of manoeu-vring the hoist that day in the hospital, springs to mind.

'How's the shower room?'

'I'll need to get in with him,' she says.

Ideally, the doors would be removed from both shower and toilet, but I imagine that's pushing it.

Regardless of how much you are prepared to pay, or how exclusive the hotel, taking Nigel away from the up-to-the-minute, customised, disabled-compatible sanctuary he enjoys at home, emphasises the degree of his disabilities.

'I'm glad you're here, Ellie.'

'Thanks. Me too.'

'Not going to be easy, is it?'

'We'll manage. We've no choice.'

Our efforts to ensure his safety and comfort are of no concern to him right now. If a wheelchair pirouettes, this is precisely what Nigel's doing. The space provided by the removal of the furniture is now his dancefloor and the iPad his servant. Nigel is no technophobe. More like a teenager than an ageing invalid. He's changing channels on the TV, flicking the lights on and off and opening and closing the blinds.

'Hey, Julie,' he says, a devilish glint in his eyes. 'We're gonna sleep in the same bed for the first time in years.'

'Don't you be getting any ideas, buggerlugs.'

Craig appears from his room along the corridor.

'Your room OK?' I ask.

'Brilliant. There's a telly in the bathroom mirror,' he says. 'How amazing is that? I've videoed it for Charlotte.'

'Not seen one before?' says Becky.

'No.'

'Bloody hell, Craig,' laughs Ellie. 'Do you ever go anywhere?'

'Yep. Cleckheaton. What's up with that?'

'Nowt, our Craig,' says Becky.

'And don't forget Emley Moor,' he adds.

'God, no. We'd never forget that Craig-y-bones,' says Ellie.

I check the time on my phone and call them to order.

'Right, you lot, listen. The doctor will be here in an hour and a half. So, unpack and shower and be back here at six-thirty. Nig, you need some time on the NIPPY while I sort stuff out.'

'OK, I stink,' says Becky, as she and Ellie slip through the adjoining door. 'I'll grab a shower, then you Ellie.'

'I'm all done,' says Craig.

'Good, you can find an English TV channel. Your dad loves to watch programmes where he doesn't understand a word when he's on holiday. Greek, maybe Spanish. Swahili, with luck.'

'Why?'

'Dunno,' says Nigel. 'I'm nuts.'

I set the NIPPY up on a side table, place the nose pillow in Nigel's nostrils and secure the strap around his head. As I switch it on, I can't resist saying. 'Admit it, you're glad you changed your mind about the doctor, aren't you?'

'Yes, you were right,' he says, his eyes closing. He'll be asleep in seconds, and Craig can watch something he understands.

The battle of the doctor was always worth the fight. In the end, my victory was a cinch. Nigel may be a stubborn old sod at times, but he's not stupid, and the strength of my argument, not to mention the skill with which it was presented, overwhelmed him. That's my interpretation, anyway. He may simply be coming to his senses. Either way, I don't care. There is no need to bundle Nigel in a taxi, senseless with fatigue and stinking like a drain. Meet with the doctor in a public place, wait for a taxi to drop us back at this hotel and repeat in the morning. The doctor is coming here, to this room, in an hour and a half. Perfect.

•••

There's a knock at precisely seven o'clock. The Swiss obsession with punctuality makes me wonder whether the doctor arrived two minutes earlier and felt compelled to stand outside and wait as the second-hand ticked by, fist at the ready, intent to bang on the door not one second before, and not one second after, seven o'clock.

I open the door to reveal a slim, tall man, dressed in a pebble-grey suit, white and grey-striped shirt and charcoal tie. He has a flat, colourless face with eyes so deeply set they're obscured by the heavy salt and pepper brows. His fair cropped hair is greying at the temples. Grey. He's overwhelmingly grey. Fortyish, I'd guess. Younger than I expected. This is the doctor who granted Nigel the provisional green light. Nigel's suicide is in this man's hands. I expected someone bearing the weight of life and death decisions to possess more experience of both.

'Mrs Casson?' he says, with a sharp German accent.

'Yes.'

'I'm the doctor. You are expecting me?'

No name? The same as Nigel's 'contact' at Dignitas. Anonymity is key. Doctor Grey, maybe?

'Please, come in.'

He shakes Nigel's hand and acknowledges Craig, Ellie and Becky, who are perched like starlings on the edge of the bed. He sits on the dining chair directly facing Nigel. I park on the other at Nigel's side. All we need is a spotlight to create an atmosphere as intimidating as Hell.

He takes a pen and clipboard, with form attached, from his briefcase. The doctor clears his throat. He fiddles with the form in the clipboard, straightens it, frees it from its clip, clips and straightens it again.

Apologising for his English, which is perfect, he says, 'Mr Casson, I must ask you some questions. Please answer truthfully.'

'Of course,' says Nigel, his voice firm. The half hour with the NIPPY has helped.

'OK. OK. OK,' says the doctor, in a halting and breathless tone. He clicks the ballpoint pen on and off a few times before writing something on the form.

I exchange glances with the starlings. We hang on his every word.

The doctor peers at Nigel. He speaks with careful concentration. 'Do you understand what it is you have requested to happen?'

'Yes.' No hesitation there, Nig.

The doctor leans back in the chair, and repeats. 'OK. OK. OK.' He presses forward again. Perhaps he's nervous. 'Do you understand what will happen if it goes ahead?'

'Yes.'

More OKs. Suppose it could be a language issue. 'OK' is international after all.

'Have you been coerced in any way in making this request?'

Nigel delivers an emphatic 'No.'

'OK. OK. OK.'

Becoming a tad irritating.

He peers at Nigel, eyebrows raised. 'Are you sure?'

'Yes.'

I've still not glimpsed those eyes. I'm guessing they'll be grey. Steel grey.

'OK,' he says, as we have come to expect.

We don't expect the meeting to be so brief, however. 'I'll come again tomorrow,' he says, standing.

'OK,' Nigel mimics, grinning. 'Thank you.'

I accompany the doctor to the door and thank him for coming.

'Is that it?' says Craig, flying from his perch.

'I thought he was going to cry,' says Becky.

'Maybe it's his first time,' says Ellie.

'Fuck me,' says Nigel. 'Not a bad hourly rate.'

Persuading Nigel to acknowledge the merits of paying for the doctor to visit us in the room is one thing, getting him to agree that it's value for money, is another.

'Drink?' I suggest.

33

ONE MORE DAY

On the morning of 24 April 2017, the incomparable panorama, portrayed with such unashamed grandiloquence in the hotel's marketing blurb, does not disappoint. The sweeping emerald carpets of the golf course are soaked in shimmering sunshine. Flags, on greens as smooth as dancefloors, scarcely flicker in the whispering breeze. The distant lake, a glistening jewel of cyan and turquoise, reflects the capacious, lush forests hugging the slopes of the giant, white-topped rocky spine of the Alps in which it nestles.

Slivers of sunlight stroke the greyness from the doctor's face as I open the door to him at precisely eleven o'clock. A hesitant smile tugs at the corners of his mouth as he takes his seat, scrutinised once again by attentive starlings. The form clasped to the clipboard doesn't require adjustment on this occasion. Ballpoint pen, tip poised and ready, mechanics of the thrust device left unchecked.

'Good morning, Doctor,' gushes Nigel.

'*Guten Morgen*, Mr Casson. How are you feeling?'

'Never better.'

The starlings, as one, roll their eyes heavenwards.

The doctor explains he must repeat yesterday's questions, to be certain nothing has occurred overnight, to trigger doubt in Nigel's mind. Should this be the case, he can halt the proceedings if he wishes.

'I understand,' says Nigel, with ear-splitting certainty.

The questions are repeated. Nigel responds with that same bold determination. The doctor mutters significantly fewer 'OKs.' There is a smattering of '*Sehr gut*,' '*Ich verstand*.'

Once completed, the doctor bundles the clipboard into his bag and bids Nigel farewell. 'I am pleased to have met with you, Mr Casson.'

'And you, Doctor.'

'I will write the prescription today,' he says.

Nigel draws a long, shuddering breath. Any concerns he harboured regarding the green light status switching from provisional to definite, are now quashed. He has passed the test. He will die tomorrow. 'Thank you very much,' he says. 'I'm so grateful.'

'Look after your family,' the doctor says as I show him out. Kind, but unnecessary.

'I will, thank you.'

Thank you? This man just signed Nigel's death warrant. And yes, those deep-set eyes are grey.

The starlings abandon their perch and gather around Nigel's chair.

'Well, that's that,' says Craig.

Nigel's rapturous face flashes like an Olympic champion's gold medal. 'Yes, fantastic, isn't it?'

'He wasn't so dreadful today, was he?' says Ellie. 'Not as nervous.'

'Still thought he was going to cry, though,' says Becky.

I take Nigel's hand in mine. 'Are you pleased with the decision, Nig?'

'Couldn't be happier.'

To ease the tension clutching my heart, I tease, 'Worth the money?'

His eyes burn into mine as he squeezes my hand. 'Every last franc.'

...

The welcoming, sun-soaked, exquisitely furnished terrace belongs to us alone. Snuggled into the Adlisberg mountain, the hotel's majestic turrets pierce the sky above us and dense forests hide an intriguing network of charming woodland walks below. In the distance, a breath-taking vista of the city of Zurich. We lounge on the lavish, deep-cushioned settees and devour a delicious lunch washed down with a divine wine.

'We should order another bottle of that,' says Nigel.

'Suits me,' says Ellie.

'And me,' affirms Becky.

'Agreed,' I say.

'I'll stick with this, ta,' says Craig, pointing to the tonic water on the table.

Perhaps we shouldn't order another bottle. Nigel hasn't drunk wine for a long time. And this is decent stuff, not cheap plonk. But it's not merely the wine we wish to savour. We want to wallow in the splendour of the surrounding scenery, soaking up the soothing rays of the sun and relish this serenity and contentment for as long as possible. So, we order another bottle. And another. Were it not for the imminent arrival of Nigel's escort, one of the two people from Dignitas who will accompany Nigel at his suicide, we would've demanded a fourth.

'Come on, drink up, you lot,' I say. 'The escort is due in half an hour. And as this is Switzerland, he won't be late.'

Ellie and Becky down the dregs of their wine with reluctance. Craig leaps to his feet. 'Why's he coming?'

'To meet Dad, I expect. It's on the itinerary. Come on Nig, let's be having you.'

He drains the last of his wine and hands me the glass. 'Have one of those sent to the room.'

As predicted, the escort is punctual. I open the door to a thin, bronzed man, around fifty years old, with a craggy, animated face and raggedy mouse-brown, rarely troubled by a brush, hair. Kind, hazel eyes twinkle and his wide smile exposes nicotine-stained teeth.

'Mrs Casson? Dignitas escort – Gabriel.'

As in angel, I think. Angel of Death, tomorrow. 'Julie. Please come in.'

He darts into the room like a cuckolded husband expecting to confront his wife's lover. A distinct whiff of tobacco comes with him. Dressed in faded denim jeans and casual baggy T-shirt with a battered leather man-bag slung over one shoulder, I envisage him tramping round India in flip-flops. The thought prompts me to examine his footwear. Jesus sandals. No socks, thank goodness.

He heads straight for Nigel and pumps his hand with the enthusiasm of a game show host.

'Mr Casson. Delighted to meet you. May I call you David?'

Nigel makes to say yes, but the last thing we need is confusion over his damn name, so I glare at him, cursing his parents, and jump in with, 'Nigel. He goes by his middle name.'

'I understand. My name is Gabriel. I will be with you tomorrow.' Each faultless English sentence bursts from his mouth like an escaping prisoner. 'We find it helps people to meet the day before,' he explains. 'Can be daunting. Better if relaxed.'

Daunting? Something of an underestimation I would say. And how could anyone be relaxed when death is imminent?

Gabriel releases Nigel's hand and focuses on each one of us with the penetrating gaze of an eagle.

'And you must be?'

'Craig.'

'Hello Craig.' A single power jerk of the hand for Craig.

'Ellie.'

'Hello Ellie.' Same.

'Becky.'

'Hello Becky.' Also, same.

'Julie.'

'Of course.' No jerk. 'You will all be present tomorrow?'

'Of course.'

Gabriel claps his hands. 'Very well.' He peers at Nigel and leans so close to him I worry he'll topple onto his knee. 'Now, Mr Casson, er, David, sorry, Nigel.'

Nigel's face is unreadable. He could be suppressing a giggle, or he could be stifling a scream. Any more intrusion into his space could prompt a claustrophobic attack. Not hanging around to find out which one it is, I grab a dining chair. 'Gabriel, here. Please sit.'

He does so. Pressing forward still, elbows on knees, fists clasped beneath his chin, he gives the impression of a coach galvanising his athlete.

'The doctor has written the prescription.'

'Excellent,' says Nigel.

Gabriel purses his lips and bobs his head, piercing eyes fixed on Nigel's. He persists with the head dipping like the Churchill insurance dog.

'You understand what this means?'

'Yes.'

I glance at the kids on the bed, motionless as statues. Wide-eyed. Alert.

Gabriel proceeds to ask similar questions as the doctor. Nigel responds with his customary self-assurance.

'Now, Nigel. How do you intend to take the barbiturate? Can you swallow?'

'Yes, but I won't take it that way,' he says.

'You must do it yourself,' insists Gabriel. 'Nobody can help you.'

Nigel lifts his T-shirt and exposes the gastric tube. 'This handy little tube should do the job,' he says.

I recall the day the tube was fitted. His body recoiling in shock as the surgeon stabbed his stomach, the gagging as the tube invaded his throat, the endless, pain-wracked night no amount of morphine could suppress. Did he endure all that for this? Was he planning this so far back?

Gabriel examines the tube. 'Excellent. Yes, we'll connect the syringe to that. Easy.'

All smiles from Nigel.

'Can you press a button?' he says.

'Yes.'

Gabriel bounds to his feet. 'Perfect. So, eleven o-clock tomorrow. I'll be waiting for you.' He pumps Nigel's hand and sprints from the room. Maybe he needs a cigarette.

'Bit different from the doctor,' I say, as I flop onto the chair vacated by Gabriel, and study my family. Craig, Ellie and Becky remain on the bed, so immersed in their thoughts they could be hypnotised. Their countenances mirror my own studiously arranged poker face. What must they be thinking? The three of them? Are they, like me, attempting to process what is happening? Are they trying to accept, after all the months of meticulous planning, the endless exchange of emails and documents, the overcoming of mounds of procedural and medical hurdles, the conquering of numerous logistical challenges, the disappointingly fruitless recce and the triumphant road trip with Mabel, that now, finally, arrangements are in place? Their dad will die tomorrow.

In contrast, the radiance flooding from Nigel's face is like a war-time beacon illuminating the darkest of nights.

'More wine anybody?' he says.

It breaks the spell. 'Yes,' chorus the girls.

'Not for me,' says Craig, diving from the bed, 'I'm bloody starving.'

'OK. Order room service,' says Nigel. 'It can be our last supper.'

'Bloody hell, Dad,' says Becky.

Ellie busies herself by emptying Nigel's catheter bag. 'You're a bugger you know.'

'And make it two bottles,' he demands.

Our elegant table, laid with crisp white linen, is soon ready, and our feast begins. *Foie gras de canard* and vichyssoise with poached quail egg and smoked salmon, displayed on the finest bone china, dished up with sparkling silver cutlery, to start. Spring lamb or beef fillet present themselves for the main, accompanied by grilled green asparagus and sweet potato mash. Chocolate mousse masquerading as an alpine mountain closes the meal. All guzzled down with the help of the glorious Swiss wine served in crystal glassware so delicate we dare not risk a clink. Not a chip or burger in sight.

Whilst the superb setting and elaborate fayre is enchanting, it is joyous laughter which seizes my attention. We could be round our rustic old kitchen table, relishing the memories. The one thing missing is Craig plonking on his keyboard.

'Do you remember moving us to Scarborough in that beaten up old pick up?' says Craig.

'All we could afford,' says Nigel.

'Still, you did end up with ten trucks and an army of scaffolders.'

'Scaffolders! You couldn't move for them,' says Ellie. 'Skiving off school was a nightmare. Couldn't go anywhere without one of your spies spotting me from on high.'

'They never blagged on you,' says Nigel.

Becky remembers the fun she and her dad had when preparing for the fitness test prior to joining the RAF. Ten press–ups before she had earned a lift to work, along with a lap of the marine drive on their bikes each morning, the waves crashing over them, the wind whipping at her frustrated tears.

'"Pedal," you said. There's me crying and covered in snot and all you ever said was "pedal."'

'Did you pass the fitness test or what?'

'Yeah, of course I did. Thanks to you.'

'How many years did you and Mum sleep on that blow up bed on the floor?' says Craig.

'Two,' I say. 'It was always flat by morning.'

'Yeah,' says Craig. 'You had to crawl round the room to sort your back out before work.'

'Stuff you do when you're skint,' says Nigel.

'You weren't skint for long though, Dad,' Ellie says.

'No,' he says. 'But busy. I thought you promised to stay five years old.'

Ellie laughs at the memory. 'Sorry, couldn't keep that one.'

'I lifted my head, and you were married. Feel like I missed it all.'

'Ah, don't be daft Dad. You more than made up for it. And anyway, I never noticed. I was too busy having fun.'

'True. Well, can't do anything about it now. What's done is done. Can't have everything and can't go back.'

'Dad,' says Craig. 'You always said: "You don't build a business sat on your arse."'

'And you don't get owt for nowt,' says Becky. 'You always said that as well.' She laughs at the memory, 'That's why you made me pay interest on the money I borrowed!'

Nigel drains the last of the wine and places his glass on the table. He inclines his chair so he's upright and rests his forearms on the table. 'I've said a lot of things,' he says. 'And I just want to say this.'

The gentle hum of the air-conditioning dissipates, as if to listen. We fall silent. Four pairs of eyes gaze into his.

'I'm so proud of you all.' The usual sluggishness of his voice also bears the slur from a generous amount of alcohol. 'I love you all very much.'

Craig wipes his nose with his serviette and clears his throat. 'We know, Dad.'

'Don't mope when I'm gone. I want you to be happy.'

Ellie bites her top lip. Becky gulps her wine.

'Look after each other, won't you? And your families.'

'Of course,' says Craig.

'Take care of your business, Craig. I'm proud of how well you've done.'

Craig picks at a bread roll. 'Thanks Dad.'

Addressing the three of them, he says, 'You do understand, don't you? I can't let MND wipe the smile from my face.'

'Yes Dad, we understand,' says Ellie. 'We know how important it is to you.'

'You pick your career back up, Ellie. And thanks for making the sacrifice to be my carer.'

'It was no sacrifice,' she says.

'You've been an absolute boon.'

Ellie glowers. 'What's a boon?'

'Something helpful. Makes a difference,' I explain.

'Oh right,' she says. 'I thought you were taking the piss, as usual, Dad.'

Nigel chuckles. 'Not a chance.'

He directs his attention to Becky. 'So, Becky. Warrant Officer on the cards?'

'Doubtful,' says Becky, scrunching her nose.

'Flight Sergeant maybe?'

'Maybe.'

'You've had a brilliant career so far. I'm proud of you. Keep pedalling.'

'I will, Dad.'

Nigel sags in his chair. The long day, emotive discussion, not to mention the wine, taking effect. Inhaling deeply, he summons the will to impart another piece of advice.

'Whatever you do, have fun. Lots of it.'

'OK, Dad.'

'And always be prepared for that kick in the bollocks.'

The sudden knock on the door jolts us away from thoughts of the future. 'Room service.'

Two waitresses, practised in the art of clearing a table without disturbing the occupants of the room, swiftly load the remnants of our meal onto a trolley. The interruption marks the end of the evening.

'Might as well call it a night, you three.' I suggest. 'I'll sort your dad.'

'You sure?' says Ellie.

'Yes, I'll manage. See you in the morning.'

...

Nigel slumps in his chair, his chin drops on his chest and mouth hangs open. A slither of drool escapes onto his T-shirt. I press him against the back of the chair and recline it until he's cradled. Floppy as a discarded condom, he doesn't protest, as I tease one arm free of his top, then the other.

'You after my body?' he slurs, T-shirt wrapped round his neck.

'How'd you guess?'

'Knew it. Can't resist me.'

'Never could, Nig.'

Swinging erratically, he tries to grab my waist, but misses.

As I slip his T-shirt over his head, glossy eyes in a lolling head somehow find mine. 'Let's get naked,' he says.

Leaning close to him I slide the sling behind his back. 'Ooo, you tease.'

This time, he doesn't miss. He wraps both arms around me and presses his face to my chest.

'I love you, Julie.'

Though muffled, the grief oozing from his words breaks my heart. 'Oh, my darling Nig,' I gasp. 'I love you too.'

'We've been happy, haven't we?'

'Incredibly.'

His flushed face is aglow with passion. 'Be happy again. When I'm gone.'

I'll never be happy again, I think. I can't conceive of life without him. 'I'll try.' I lie.

'Remember the fab times,' he says. 'Sorry MND fucked it up.'

Didn't it though?

I cup his face in my hands and plant a kiss on his nose. 'Now you, don't be getting all maudlin.'

'Sorry,' he mumbles, face still pressed to my chest. 'And one more thing.'

'What's that?'

'Don't forget to brush Bodger.'

'You daft sod,' I say, tucking the sling beneath his legs, ready for the hoist. 'I won't forget. Anyway, do you still want to sleep in the bed? Or your chair?'

A smirk spreads across his face and Lucifer knocks out an award-winning jive from the depths of his wine-soaked eyes. Hammered he may be. Dead he isn't. 'Bed.'

We've not slept in the same bed for years. Not slept in the same room. On this, our final night, we need to hold each other again. We yearn to lie beside one another on this cavernous bed, feel our bodies close together, and fall asleep, hand in hand. Nothing more.

I suspect the hotel doesn't possess enough pillows to bolster Nigel on the bed. Regardless, I replicate the shape of his profiling mattress. Three to support his head, two beneath his shoulders, one under each arm. Let's give it a shot. By the time I attach the sling to the hoist and lift him from his chair, Nigel is slipping into oblivion. Like a comatose orangutan his head flops forward and his arms dangle at his sides.

I suppose it was always a mad idea. The pillows scatter as I lower him, and he slips between them as surely as a salmon off a rock. Lying flat, unable to move, without the assurance of a control in his hand to raise him up and down, panic replaces the passion in his eyes, and he barks like a distressed walrus. No amount of pillow plumping will fix this. Indeed, walking on water would present fewer challenges.

Giving up, I raise him from the bed and secure him in his chair.

'Goodnight, my darling,' I whisper, kissing the cheek of my already snoring husband. I cover him with a sheet, climb on the empty bed and watch him sleep.

Oh Nig, we've had such a lovely day. A perfect day, even. Just blown it by drinking too much. Hell, we're not strangers to booze on a normal day, and this is no normal day. Who wouldn't get drunk the night before they die? Like a condemned man, Nig, were you relishing your last ever drop of an exceptional vintage? Raising a glass to your life? Saying farewell? For weeks you've had to say goodbye to people you love. Tomorrow you'll say goodbye to us. Was today, my darling, just for you?

Or was it something more? Were you hoping to quash your nerves? Your fears? Scare away the demons and banish any doubts you might have? No. Never. You've talked about nothing else for months. You have no doubts. This is what you want. But even you could be scared. Bravery is not the absence of fear, they say, and you, Nig, are the bravest man I will ever know.

I climb from the bed and pour the last of the wine into my glass.

Well, I'm bloody scared. I need you, Nig. I cannot conceive how immense will be the gap in my life when you've left it. Forty-three years we've been together. You, the one person in the world who has shared my most painful and joyful moments. You know everything about me and love me anyway. You know what I'm thinking without the need for me to utter a single word. You pick me up when I fall, you hold me close and keep me safe. And you'll be gone in the morning.

I can't be alone tonight. I drain my glass and stand up. Gently, I inch Nigel's chair as close to the edge of the bed as I can get it. I needn't be so cautious. I could charge him down the M62 and it wouldn't wake him. Once in position, I clamber onto the bed and lie beside him and reach for his hand. It's a little awkward. Blessed sleep will be harder to find than usual, but I don't care.

'We will hold hands tonight, my love, as we'd planned,' I whisper. 'Because tomorrow, you'll leave me, forever.'

My lips stroke the delicate, translucent skin on the back of his hand. 'And I love you too much to stop you.'

34

NIGEL'S CURE

25 April 2017

Thousands of pins pricking the back of my retinas force my stinging eyelids open. I feel like I nodded off seconds ago.

Nigel, already awake and engaged, as usual, with the virtual world provided by his iPad, inclines his head and grunts. 'You look rough.'

I spring from the bed pretending nothing in my body hurts. 'Morning to you too. How are you feeling, mister "order another bottle of wine?"'

'I'm great.'

'No tramp's sock in your gob?'

'No.'

'Bloody hell, my mouth is festering. I'll clean my teeth before I inflict a kiss.'

'More like his jockstrap,' he chuckles, as I dash to the bathroom.

Once the menace of morning breath is eliminated, Nigel's catheter bag emptied, the room's 'do everything with this iPad' discarded in favour of opening the blinds the old-fashioned way, and the magnitude of this unimaginably difficult day ahead besieging my consciousness, I cup Nigel's face in my hands and ask, 'How are you? Are you nervous?'

'Not at all.'

I search his face for signs of apprehension, the faintest flicker of doubt. There are none. 'Are you sure you want to do this, Nig?'

'Definitely. It's the right thing to do.' No hesitation there.

'You're tremendous. You know that?'

'I like to think so,' he says, pursing his lips to receive a kiss.

A knock on the door heralds the arrival of room service and Craig, lured like a puppy in pursuit of a string of pork sausages, follows the waitress into the room. Ellie and Becky appear through the adjoining door, and each demolish a long glass of freshly squeezed orange juice before the food is transferred from trolley to table.

'Thirsty?'

Two pairs of beetroot-shadowed bloodshot eyes blink back at me.

'A change in the weather,' says Nigel congenially, to our waitress, as she places a bowl of fruit and a platter of meat and cheese on the table. Please don't ask her where she's from, Nig.

'Yes,' she says. 'Swiss weather is like a girl's mood. Always changing.'

'You're not kidding,' says Craig. 'The sky's got a right monk on.'

The breath-taking scenery outside our window is denied us today. Thick, black clouds churn ominously in a glowering sky, jostling like squabbling siblings in a spiteful bid to mask the majesty of the mountains. Suffocating smog smothers the lush carpets of the fairways like a miserable shroud. The gloom mirrors the inside of my head.

'The sky's crying. It's sad,' says Ellie, kissing her dad's head. 'No sunshine allowed today.'

The scrumptious breakfast, displayed before us, deserves to be devoured whilst accompanied by the soundtrack of jovial chitchat. Cereals scream for a splash of milk; bacon begs to be paired with sausage, egg and grilled tomatoes; breads await the enlivening addition of meat and cheese, and the cocktail of fruit entices like gleaming gems. Yet the family who, only yesterday, lingered for hours around this table, with appetites insatiable for delicious food, fine wine, heart-rending memories and joyous laughter, now dwell in uneasy silence, occasionally meeting the worried eyes of another and barely touching the banquet before us. Craig makes a valiant attempt at a sausage, the girls chase a few berries around a bowl, Nigel nibbles on a bit of cheese and I chew on a chunk of bread. The orange juice and lemon tea are, however, consumed with gusto, by all except Craig, who has no need to wrestle a hangover.

'Nobody hungry?' I ask.

'Can't swallow it,' says Becky, dropping her spoon.

Ellie and Craig end the pretence of forcing food in their faces and thrust their plates away as if the milk would sour, and the cheese curdle, the second they hit their bellies.

'Feel a bit sick. Must be the wine,' says Nigel. 'Can't be covered in vom when I croak.'

'Lovely image,' I say, ditching my chunk of bread. My own delicate stomach churning like an off-balance washing machine on a spin cycle. I'm not convinced it's simply the wine making him feel sick. Perhaps he is the tiniest bit anxious after all?

'Would you mind giving me a shower, Ellie?' Nigel asks. 'It relaxes me.'

'Of course, Dad.'

Grateful for the excuse, we scramble from the table.

'I'll go change,' says Craig.

'I'll paint my face,' says Becky.

'I'll organise your clothes, Nig.'

Nigel, in control of the minute details of his final day, has already chosen his T-shirt. A comfortable pale grey number with the words 'Made in England' monogrammed on the front. I suspect he wishes to emphasise the point, as he is forced to die elsewhere. '1954', signifying the year of his birth, is written beneath those words.

He emerges from the shower, bundled like a baby in fluffy white towels, his face pink and smiling.

'Will you dress him?' says Ellie, standing by his chair, vest top and leggings dripping wet, a puddle of water forming at her feet.

'Been for a swim?' I ask.

'I had to squeeze in with him.'

'Thanks again, Ellie,' says Nigel. 'You've been brilliant.'

Hands on hips, the puddle now a lake, she grins at him. 'A boon, by any chance?'

'Yes. A massive boon.'

...

On any other occasion, the seductive splendour of the Dolder Grand lobby would induce a sense of wonder. The magnificent bronze goddess, in the heart of this exquisite foyer, peers at us mortals from the ornate column upon which she stands. The immense shimmering chandelier above her illuminates the marble-clad walls with masses of glittering, dancing diamonds. Palatial staircases sweep elegantly to the gallery above, where the grand, lofty ceiling is framed with elaborate cornices.

I don't see any of it. All I can see is the concierge behind his desk. He ordered our taxis yesterday. He was attentive and professional. I handed him the address, which is in the village of Pfaffikon – the one next to Uster – printed in bold to avoid confusion as there are two Pfaffikons. Fancy rocking up at the wrong one. Unlikely, given the vigilance of Nigel's anonymous Dignitas contact and his or her precise instructions. Wheelchair accessible taxis are not common in Zurich, the concierge tells me. They need to be booked well in advance.

He catches me staring at him. 'I'll let you know when the taxis arrive,' he says, before resuming his task. Does he know where we're headed? Is he aware Pfaffikon is home to Dignitas? Has he figured out our plan? An ill, disabled man, here in Zurich, with his family? I press a fist to my brow and rattle my head in a bid to dispel the nonsense lurking within it. Stop being ridiculous, Julie. Surely disabled people visit Zurich without intending to kill themselves. Still, what will he surmise when four, not five of us return?

'I don't bloody believe you, Dad,' says Craig, providing my baloney-ridden brain with a welcome distraction.

'What?' says Nigel.

'You're checking the bank? Today? Now? Mum, he's checking the bank.'

'Yeah,' I shrug. 'It's what he does.'

'Every day,' he says. 'Take the iPad now, Julie. I'm finished.'

I release the iPad from its clamp and stuff it in my bag. This piece of technology has been Nigel's lifeline, his gateway to the world, for years: the means to communicate and be involved, to contribute to discussions; to share his playlist late into the night with revellers dancing around his bed; to impose his jokes on unsuspecting Facebook friends and to play poker with like-minded gamblers. And, of course, to keep a grip on his finances. Now, all that is over. He has no further need of it. His final hours are for us alone.

'We should take a selfie?' he says. 'Our last family photo.'

I join the kids in gathering around his chair. 'Fine idea.'

'I'll take it,' says Becky, grabbing her phone.

'Are your arms long enough?' says Craig, as Becky raises her phone.

'Yes, we're all in.'

'Don't make me look fat,' says Ellie.

'Say bollocks,' says Nigel.

There it is, our final family photograph. Five smiling faces, none so jubilant as Nigel's, captured in Zurich's most luxurious hotel lobby, give the impression of a family heading off on a thrilling day out. And they say photographs never lie.

'Your taxis are here, Madam,' says the concierge.

'Let's do this,' says Nigel, racing for the door.

Once Craig and the driver succeed in ramming Nigel's extra-large wheelchair into the pocket sized, not unlike an adapted Reliant Robin, taxi, and strap him in so tightly I fear the tube he will need within the hour will be crushed, I squeeze into the front seat and hand our driver the prepared, no-room-for-error post-card, bearing the address of our destination. In contrast, Craig, Ellie and Becky, furnished with similar destination instructions, travel ahead in a high-performance Merc.

We leave the Dolder Grand and make our way down the hill. The rain has washed the roads to a glossy sheen whilst the ghostly silhouettes on the edge of the woodland remain veiled in mist until we pass so close, we glimpse the leaves drooping under the weight of the droplets. Or tears, if you buy into Ellie's notion the sky is crying.

English is not one of the languages spoken by our driver, but this doesn't prevent him from jabbering away in some, or possibly all four, commonly spoken languages in Switzerland. I recognise the word *'physiotherapie'* and gather, due to his insistent prodding of the postcard, the address given to us by Dignitas was once a physiotherapy studio. This knowledge, combined with his wheel-chair-bound passenger, has prompted him to put two and two together and come up with five. I'm not prepared to burst that bubble.

'Sehen! Sehen!' cries our vivacious driver, pointing to the skies above us as a united formation of jets sweep in a dramatic arc, right in front of the car.

'Militärisch übung,' he gushes, which I guess means military training.

'Did you see that, Nig?'

'Yes,' he says. 'Just like the Red Arrows over Tyne Bridge when me and Mel did the Great North Run.'

'Exactly. They're saluting you.' I say.

The rain dwindles to a drizzle as we leave the main road and drive into what appears to be an industrial estate. We pass an electrical hardware store, a vast, rectangular warehouse, a decorators' merchants and a Lidl supermarket on the corner, before we come to a halt outside a featureless two-storey, box of a building, with a cladded blue exterior. Is this it? Amid ordinary workplaces? With people milling around? Does anyone ever speculate, as they pop into Lidl to do their weekly shop, what happens at the blue house? Who could dream such extraordinary activity could occur in such an ordinary setting? But yes, this must be the place. Craig, Ellie and

Becky are already out of their car, and I notice Gabriel standing by the hedge at the front of the unit. What did I expect? A neon light flashing 'Dignitas. The Dying Room?' Gabriel flicks a cigarette end into a bush and waves.

Nigel slides from the taxi so smoothly I marvel at the fuss shoving him in. I pay the driver the 110-franc fare, and he hands me his business card, gesturing for me to call for the return journey. Another bubble I won't be bursting.

'Did you clock the jets?' asks Craig.

'Yes, impressive.'

'We thought it was just for you, Dad,' he says.

'Same here,' I say.

'Mr Casson. Nigel,' cries Gabriel, grasping Nigel's hand. 'Excellent to see you.'

He guides us along the short path to the door, past a slatted wooden bench where, judging from the soggy pile of tab ends in the ashtray on the seat, is where Gabriel spends considerable time.

'Come. This way,' he says, as courteous as a host welcoming guests for lunch.

A ramp provides easy access for Nigel, and we enter a dimly lit, square-shaped room. The blinds at the windows are half-closed – against prying eyes – I assume, and additional light is provided by two old-fashioned shaded standard lamps. Despite innumerable references in the media to the Dignitas 'clinic', there is nothing remotely clinical about it. It couldn't be considered stylish, either. The furniture is basic, functional and unquestionably cheap. A compact two-seater settee and chairs, covered in a fabric evoking memories of my grandma's parlour, are grouped next to a teak coffee table bearing a jug of water, drinking glasses, a ceramic vase holding a bunch of weary tulips and a selection of Swiss chocolates. A thoughtful addition, the chocolates – the barbiturate tastes vile, I understand. There is also an opened box of tissues. Can't imagine why. Against the wall is a hospital bed covered in a single sheet. A gilt-framed picture of the Alps hangs above it. The far wall is occupied by a circular wooden dining table, upon which is an A4 envelope pocket file and a box containing a gadget topped with a large red button and a tube. Four ladder-back chairs, one of which has Gabriel's brown leather man-bag slung over it, surround the table. The place is reminiscent of a budget holiday rental.

'Meet Anna, my colleague,' says Gabriel, as a lavender-grey-haired lady emerges from what is obviously a kitchen.

How do you recruit for this job? I ponder, as I mutter my hello to Anna. What would make you choose to apply? Dressed like a relic from the 1950s in a pale blue twinset and A-line skirt, she would appear more at home at, well, home. Or maybe on the bakery counter at the Lidl on the corner.

'May I offer you a cup of tea? Coffee?' she asks, in a voice as subdued as Gabriel's is fervent.

We are all, except Nigel, caught off guard. Craig, Ellie and Becky gape at her like she's just proposed we all snort coke. The unexpected conventions of polite hospitality, as if we've popped in for afternoon tea and a jolly natter, seem absurd. Nigel, who is entirely at ease, signals 'no thank you', and Craig and the girls recover enough to do the same.

'Coffee, please. Black, no sugar.' I say, not wishing to be rude.

It's beyond peculiar.

Gabriel invites us to sit. We poise on the edge of the seats, upright and rigid. I focus on Craig, Ellie and Becky, compelling my gaze alone, as not a single word will emerge from my mouth, to comfort them with, 'We'll get through this. We'll be OK. We have each other.' Nigel locates himself in the centre of the room. He grins, raises his eyebrows, eyes wide and sparkling with mischief, pulls the kind of face you pull when you've done something naughty, like fart in a lift.

'OK,' says Gabriel, spreading his arms aloft, palms forward, index fingers pointing upwards. 'This is what is to happen.' An image of the Pope blessing the masses in St Peter's Square romps into my mind.

Anna places my coffee on the table. I ignore it. She stands against the wall, hands clasped beneath her chin, observing the scene over frameless spectacles. The scene strikes me as rehearsed. It always happens this way. Gabriel does the talking while she ensures nothing is missed.

'Paperwork first. Nigel, can you sign your name?'

'Yes.'

'A mark will do.'

'No, I'll sign.'

Gabriel grips Nigel's shoulders and fixes him with a penetrative stare. He enunciates each word, with exaggerated care. 'Nigel, you can still change your mind. Do you wish to go ahead?'

'Yes.'

As predicted. All hopes of a change of heart were dashed earlier this morning. I glance at our son and daughters and press a consoling expression on my face. As one, their stiff shoulders sag a little.

'OK,' says Gabriel, stepping back. 'The anti-emetic drug will be administered through your tube, via a syringe. This stops you from being sick when you take the barbiturate.'

'That's good,' says Nigel, perhaps regretting not having a spot of breakfast after all.

'Anna and I will leave you to spend time alone with your family for twenty minutes, while the anti-emetic takes effect. We will stay in the other room. Give you privacy.'

'Thank you.'

'Some like to play music. Bluetooth your favourite tunes to the speaker on the table.'

'Perfect,' says Nigel, smiling in our direction. Which bonkers, inappropriate tune will he choose, I wonder?

'Everything clear?' says Gabriel, addressing the room.

We nod like respectful students, as if we had been issued with the housekeeping instructions for the fire exits and loos.

Gabriel takes a pile of papers out of the A4 envelope file. 'Finally, Nigel. I must tell you exactly what will occur.'

We press forward once more. As alert as gazelles surrounded by lions.

'Are you sure you wish to do this today?'

'Yes,' says Nigel, his voice as formidable as I've ever heard it.

'Do you understand what will happen?'

'Yes.'

'After a few minutes, you will fall asleep. You will not wake up.'

'Yes.'

'It always works. It has never failed.'

'Good.'

'Is this what you want?'

'Definitely.'

His resolve is like a punch to my chest, and I release the breath I'm holding in a gasp. Craig's and the girls' shoulders droop still more and one by one they shrink into their chairs. Our gaze locks. 'Be strong. For Dad. We can do this.' I scream, in silence.

Nigel grasps the pen in a trembling hand. He could so easily have scribbled a simple mark, but no, he paints a meticulous, flourishing signature on the swathe of documents handed to him. One of them grants Dignitas power of attorney. This enables them to certify his death and arrange the removal of his body for cremation. Another, 'Declaration of Suicide' confirms Nigel has voluntarily committed suicide and has been thoroughly informed by Dignitas of the process.

...

Gabriel dispenses the anti-emetic into Nigel's tube. This is it. It's happening.

'Call us when you're ready,' he says as he and Anna retreat to the kitchen.

We regard each other, steadily. Quietly. Each one of us processing this uniquely taxing situation, unsure what to say or do. I'm aware of the swish of a passing car on the rain-soaked road, the whistle of a kettle coming to a boil in the kitchen. The juddering of my heart.

'Chocolate anyone?' I mutter, like an imbecile. There are times when saying anything to fill the silence, instead of nothing, is a mistake. This is one of those times. Nobody wants a bloody chocolate.

'What about some music?' says Nigel.

'OK,' says Craig. 'What would you like?'

'Enigma?'

'That's all we need,' Craig groans. 'Couldn't you come up with something a bit more mournful?'

Could be worse. Nigel could have requested *Staying Alive* by the Bee Gees or Queen's *Another One Bites the Dust*. This, at least, feels appropriate for the moment. Ellie selects Enigma on her phone and sends it to the speaker. Moments later, the poignant strains of *Sadeness* fill the room.

This is our time. Now.

Craig approaches first. He stands tall, his shoulders square and strong. His jaw clenched so tightly the veins in his neck bulge purple. 'Bye Dad,' he chokes.

Nigel opens his arms and Craig collapses into his embrace.

'Goodbye, son,' he says.

After a moment, Craig stands and grips Nigel's hand in both of his. 'You'll always be my hero, Dad. You always were.'

'Thank you, Craig. That's lovely.'

'Well done,' I whisper, as Craig makes way for Ellie.

Tears pooling in her eyes, Ellie kisses her dad on his cheek and, voice trembling, says, 'I'll miss you, Dad. You were always there for me, you know. And in my head and my heart, you always will be.'

He folds her in his arms. 'I know darling. Goodbye.'

'Bless you,' I say, pressing a tissue into her hand.

Becky wraps herself around her dad's shoulders, smothering her tears by burying her face in his neck.

'Bye Dad,' she weeps.

'Bye, sweetheart.'

Strangling her sobs, she rubs at her eyes and takes a deep breath. She bends and plants a kiss on his brow and rests her palm against his cheek. 'You can stop pedalling now, Dad,' she says.

She is rewarded with the sunniest of smiles and an extra hug. 'Thank you, Becky. I will. But you can't.'

'Perfect,' I whisper, as she joins her siblings behind Nigel's chair.

Standing there, the three of them, composed now, their emotions once again under control, I am staggered by their courage and resilience.

'I'm so proud of you all,' I say. 'You're a credit to me and your dad.'

'Here, here,' says Nigel.

He holds out his hand for me. As I peer into those fathomless pools, I know I will never again see or feel, for as long as I live, such overwhelming and unconditional love.

'It's been a joy to be your husband, Julie. You've made me very happy.'

My heart heaves in my chest and the clenching of my throat makes me dizzy. Already on fire from battling to restrain obstinate tears, I close my traitorous eyes and visualise our three children, who, moments ago, said their last goodbyes.

Don't. You. Dare. Cry.

I don't recognise my own quivering voice as I compel the words, 'You've made me happy too. I'll miss you, Nig.'

He draws me towards him, and I rest my face close to his. 'In the words of the song,' he says, 'I will always love you.'

I brush my lips with his and drop a kiss on each eyelid. 'I love you, Nig.'

'I know. Look after our family.'

'I will.'

He relaxes into his chair and grins, that rascally glimmer returning to his eyes, 'Stroke Bodger for me, and –'

'Don't forget to brush him,' I interject. 'I won't.'

'I'm ready,' he says. 'Let Gabriel and Anna back in.'

Ellie silences Enigma's *'Gravity of Love'* as the escorts enter the room. Gabriel takes the red buttoned gadget from the box, attaches a syringe bearing the lethal barbiturate and places it on the bed, within Nigel's reach. He fits the cylinder into Nigel's gastric tube and climbs onto the bed, where Anna is already seated.

Once more, like unwilling participants dragged in to witness a macabre ceremony, we balance on the edge of our seats, stiff backed and silent.

'When you're ready Nigel, press the red button.'

He glances in our direction and snickers, 'I've always wanted to press the red button.'

'Ready?' says Gabriel.

'Ready.'

I'm aware of our children's pulsating hearts, as well as my own.

'Oh, wait,' Nigel says, hand hovering above the button. 'I need a penny to pay the ferryman.'

'Ferryman?' says Gabriel.

'Yes, to cross the river Styx.'

Ellie, Becky and I dive into our bags in search of a purse. Craig rummages in his pockets. What are the chances of any one of us having a penny?

'Of course!' cries Gabriel, leaping from the bed. 'Yes, here. Look, I have some English coins.'

Nigel accepts a coin: a pound, not a penny. Still, it's a fair bet the ferryman has increased his fare over the centuries. He curls his fingers around it.

'Right. Go for it,' he says.

With not a second's hesitation, a cheeky grin creasing his face, he presses the button. I grip Ellie's and Becky's hands, Becky clutches Craig's. Unable to move, not daring to breathe, we stare as the contraption closes the syringe and pushes the barbiturate into Nigel's body. Once the syringe empties and Gabriel removes the tube connected to Nigel, we scramble to our feet and rush to enfold him in our arms.

We have moments left.

'I love you, darling,' I whisper, as I kiss his cheek.

'Love you,' he murmurs.

Through my tears, I gaze, for the final time, into those eyes. There is no sadness there, no fear. There is resolve, acceptance, and love.

'Be happy, Julie.'

One more kiss.

'I'm feeling sleepy.'

Then, the ultimate, mesmerising, unforgettable smile.

We cling to him as he slips into a state of unconsciousness. We embrace him when his breathing grows heavy. We won't abandon him when the room reverberates with his rumbling snore, the harrowing echo of his descent into a fatal coma. As his body slumps and his grip on the ferryman's coin loosens, still, we cling to him. When the sporadic rasp of his breathing fades to a muted hush, when the soft whisper of his breath is no more, and when we are consumed by a suffocating, deadening silence, we continue to hold him.

The only man I will ever love, is dead.

Gabriel approaches and places a hand on my shoulder. 'I'm sorry,' he murmurs. 'It's time.'

We can't let go. Can't move.

'I'm sorry,' he insists.

He's asking us to leave. To desert him. To walk away and forsake him. To discard him here, in this shitty room, with two strangers and a vase of wilting tulips.

Gabriel opens the door. 'Please. It's been too long. A taxi is waiting.'

Craig helps his sisters prize themselves away. He cradles them as they stumble towards the door.

Before I step away from Nigel's body, I tighten his fingers around the ferryman's coin and kiss his hand. This, his final act of control, to ensure his passage from this life to the next.

'Travel safely across the river Styx, my darling.'

35

NIGEL'S LAST GOODBYE

If the sky was gently weeping when we delivered Nigel to the Dignitas house, it now rages with convulsive sobs. The pelting rain batters the taxi roof, and the frantic swish of the wipers struggles to compete with the ferocious downpour. Rivers of water cascade across the windows in a wriggling frenzy, to be whipped up and swamped by yet more angry torrents.

Is this you Nig? Is this your fury? Are you floundering on the banks of the river Styx? Is it too stormy to cross? Should I have begged you to stay? If not for me, for them? I glance at Craig, Ellie and Becky. Not a word has been spoken since we clambered into the car. Each one, alone with their thoughts, stares sightlessly through the taxi windows. Craig glowers at the rain, his handsome face creased with loss. Ellie, snuffling and biting the back of her hand, presses her head against the cold glass, and a single tear trickles unchecked down the curve of Becky's cheek. Oh Nig, what have you done? What have I let you do? How do I help them through this?

I turn from their pain and close my eyes. The final image of Nigel floods my mind: the sad, drooping mouth, the purplish hue of his skin, his body slumped and awkward in his chair, his loosening grip on the ferryman's coin.

I wonder what's happening now. Is Gabriel smoking a fag while Anna does the washing up? Have the police arrived? What if something isn't right? What if something's missing from the paperwork? Will they turn up at the hotel? Then what?

As we arrive at the Dolder Grand, I can't help but scour the car park for a police car. There is none. Nevertheless, we charge like fleeing criminals to the main door and into the security of the sumptuous lobby.

'Let's get to my room,' I say.

The concierge looks up from the desk and smiles. I ignore him and continue to bound towards the stairs like it's raining as heavily inside as it is out. I don't want to witness his puzzled expression as he peers at the door, expecting the pleasant gentleman in the wheelchair to enter. I can't watch him search for another taxi approaching. I can't bear to observe the questions flitting across his face: perhaps he's visiting someone? Probably has an appointment and will be back later? They haven't forgotten him, surely? Ah, then comes the realisation. Pfaffikon? The taxi's destination this morning. Yes. Of course. Dignitas.

The room is exactly as we left it a little over an hour ago, but it seems as vast and desolate as a long-abandoned mausoleum. Our footsteps intrude into the space and disturb the silence. The mobile hoist looms like an accusing sentinel. Am I no longer needed? Have you no further use of me? The sling, so old it's ingrained with his skin and smudged with his sweat, is draped across it. I resist the temptation to bury my face in the fabric. The NIPPY, nose pillow still attached, haunts the table, awaiting its user. I swear I can hear its rhythmical whoosh as it breathes. Crumpled towels litter the shower room floor and the distinctive aroma of his favourite after-shave – Paco Rabanne – lingers in the air. I almost expect him to whirl in and demand a cuppa. But that won't happen, will it?

Craig pushes the hoist aside and the three of them sink onto the edge of the bed.

'How are you doing?' I ask. 'OK?'

'Yeah,' they croak, their voices as husky as a reluctant morning grunt following a heavy night.

'Shall I order room service?'

'Could do with a tea,' says Craig.

No matter how terrible the ordeal, the humble cup of tea will always provide a modicum of comfort.

'Wine?' suggests Ellie.

Wine too. That's comforting.

'Maybe a coffee,' adds Becky.

'I'll order all three.'

I glance at the clock on my phone.

'We need to let people know. They'll be anxious. They might be wondering if your dad went through with it. Hoping he didn't.'

'Never any chance of that,' says Craig. 'Anybody who knew him would be certain he'd go through with it.'

'I suppose you're right,' I sigh. 'I've asked him every day since September if he had any doubts –'

'No way,' says Ellie. 'Remember when we were all together shortly after his diagnosis? He mentioned Dignitas back then. I think it was always his plan.'

'Yes, he did. But he never mentioned it again, did he? Until he was ready.'

'It's what he wanted, Mum,' says Becky. 'That was obvious. We need to be happy for him.'

Looking at our children's grief-stricken faces, I can't believe happiness will ever light up their countenances again.

'You're not angry with him? For leaving us?'

'Not at all,' insists Becky. 'I'm so glad he could do this. On his own terms.'

'Exactly,' says Ellie. 'Just wish he could have done it at home.'

'Yes. Thing is,' says Craig, his voice quivering, 'he would have lived longer. A year, maybe two? He needn't have gone yet.'

My heart clogs my throat as I open my arms to embrace them. 'Come here, kids. We still have each other.'

I hold them until room service knocks on the door.

'Hello again,' chirrups the young waitress who brought breakfast this morning. She guides the trolley to the table and prepares to unload it.

'Leave the trolley, please,' I say. 'We'll do it, thank you.'

'Of course,' she says, smiling as she meets my gaze.

Will she notice our blotchy faces and swollen, red-rimmed eyes? Is she looking for the man in the wheelchair: the nice man who chatted about the weather this morning? Will she mention his absence to her colleagues? The concierge?

'He went out this morning and never came back,' he'll say, furtively tapping his nose. 'Not for me to speculate, but I have my suspicions.'

I banish from my mind the vision of the hotel staff gossiping below stairs like the servants in *Downton Abbey* and pour the drinks.

'Come on. Let's make our phone calls.'

Craig takes his tea to his room where he will contact Charlotte, in private. The girls head next door, to telephone Danny and Daz. A bottle of wine goes with them. It falls to me to inform first Melanie, then Paula. They are the ones elected to spread the news to family and friends. I welcome the time alone and take a moment to gather my thoughts and gaze out of the window. The driving rain has dwindled to a drizzle but the bleak, impenetrable mist shrouds the golf course and mountains in a blanket of misery. I take long deep breaths, exhaling slowly as I try to recall the controlled breathing technique from the one occasion I practised yoga.

It's time.

Melanie answers instantly. I picture her, clutching her phone. Les, Tracey, Derek and Sally on the edge of their seats, desperate to hear, yet dreading the news that will shatter their hearts.

'Hello?' Her voice is contained and resolute. I can feel the tightness in her neck as she holds it together.

My breath bubbles in my throat. A tremulous squeak escapes. 'He's gone.'

I hear her gasp as the tension bursts from her body. I sense her shoulders sag and her face crumple.

'Just before noon,' I stutter. 'Swiss time.'

I know the time Nigel died will be significant. The five of them had arranged to spend the morning on Holy Island, about an hour's drive from Mel and Derek's Newcastle home, to lay flowers in a simple ceremony to say goodbye. Perhaps that was precisely the time the sea claimed the bouquet, or the rain stopped pouring and the sun appeared from behind the clouds? Sometimes the sky performs fanciful stunts at times of death. Or had they already returned to Newcastle, and this was the point they clinked glasses in salute of their brother? The waiting to hear must have been agonising. What will be happening now? Will he change his mind?

'How are you all?' she chokes.

Craig's, Ellie's and Becky's traumatised expressions, on the way back in the taxi, swamp my mind. I recall their immense bravery as they exchanged those final, loving words, their unwavering support for their dad's actions and their conviction that what he did was right. Even so, I know the three of them, like me, are plagued by a new and suffocating sorrow. Whilst we can acknowledge that his suffering is over, nothing can stem the sadness that he had to suffer in the first place. People will assure us that time will help us manage our despair, and we will learn to carry our grief, rather than be crushed beneath its weight. But not yet. Not now.

'I can't talk,' I stammer.

'That's OK,' she says, her voice breaking. 'Talk later. Love to you all.'

We end the call. I pour a glass of wine. They'll collapse into one another's arms now and seek comfort. Then, once composed, each will share the news with their own children, wider family members and circle of personal friends. For those who are expecting the call, it will end their anxious wait, but for many, it will be a dreadful shock.

Paula next.

The phone rings and rings. I know exactly what she'll be doing. She'll be sitting up in bed, where she will have spent the morning. She'll stare at the phone as Tom holds it towards her. Frozen. Not daring to hear the news.

'It's Julie,' Tom will say.

'I know.'

'Answer it.'

At last, I hear a plaintive, 'Julie?'

The wretchedness engulfed in that single word smashes my resolve and my own voice betrays me. I save us both the need to talk further by gushing, 'He's gone. We're OK. Sorry, can't talk. Love you.'

I fall onto the bed and stuff my face into a pillow, smothering my sobs in its melting softness and I imagine Paula doing the same. Once her tears are spent, she'll drag herself out of bed and phone our brothers Nigel and Jez. They'll ask how I'm doing, and she'll say, 'She's OK, but she can't talk.' Then she'll text Glyn and Gamby. In turn, Glyn will inform all the lads at DNC Scaffolding and Gamby will spread the word at the golf club. She'll contact Graham and Bruce and those few friends who know what's happening today. Paula and Tom will then drive to Mum's and stay and console her for a while.

And so, the news will ripple ever outward until all family members and friends are aware of Nigel's death. The knowledge that this was happening won't diminish their grief. They'll empathise with us and bemoan the tragedy of our enforced flight to Switzerland. They'll ask if there's anything they can do to help. Probably arrange for a bouquet of flowers to be delivered. As people do, they'll search for the mercy in his death. He took control, they'll say. Did what he had to do. His suffering is over. They may wonder if, should they ever be faced with such a choice, they would have the courage to do the same. They will pray never to be confronted with that dilemma.

Craig enters the room. The misery scored into his face adds years to his appearance. He pours himself a fresh cup of tea.

'How did it go? How was Charlotte?'

'Sad. Sends her love.'

'The girls?'

'Quiet. Don't know how to deal with it.'

'I'm sure they don't.'

'Charlotte's kept them off school.'

'Bless them.'

Ellie and Becky appear through the adjoining door, clutching full wine glasses and an empty bottle. Ellie drags her feet as though being led to the scaffold for execution, she slumps onto the bed and gulps a mouthful of wine.

'Was that awful?' I say.

Her voice is heavy with longing as she says, 'Yeah. Ben and Tom are not doing very well.'

'Poor darlings.'

'Danny's going to take them out for tea. Try and help them through it.'

My heart aches as I look at these three exceptional people. I know how vital it's been for me to have them here with me: to share their pain, to give them solace. Craig and Ellie must be desperate to hold their children. Making this journey with Nigel is one thing, but the agony of separation from their own families is unimaginable.

'What about you Becky, love. How's Daz?'

Tears pool in Becky's eyes as she glances up from her wine. 'He's coping. He got the train to Scarborough once he dropped off the motorhome.'

'How'd that go?' says Craig. 'Did she ask why it was returned so early?'

'Yes.'

She pauses. We wait for her to continue.

'And?' says Ellie.

'He broke down,' chokes Becky. 'And he told her.'

'Oh, poor Daz,' I say.

Ellie gasps. 'Shit. What did she say?'

'She doesn't blame us. Completely agrees.'

'Bloody hell,' says Craig. 'That's good.'

'Yeah,' says Becky, extending her glass for me to fill. 'He's going to see Danny this afternoon.'

'Good. Wine, Ellie?'

'Yes.'

'Craig. More tea?'

'No. It'll be cold.'

Glasses filled, composure restored, there is one final task to complete.

I have always excelled at mentally putting things in boxes. Now is the time to arrange the delicate slivers of my shattered mind into their own virtual compartments, to be brought out when I am ready to deal with that splinter of pain. Into one box goes my yearning to be with our loved ones at home. There is a box for my grandchildren, sons-in-law and daughter-in-law, another for Nigel's siblings and partners, one for my own siblings and partners and finally my Mum. I can't share their torment right now. File it. Getting these three through the next forty-eight hours is my greatest concern.

'OK kids. One more job to do for your dad. It's time to put your dad's final post on Facebook.'

I retrieve Nigel's iPad from my bag and sit at the desk. Craig, Ellie and Becky gather behind me. I find his Facebook account and paste the post he so thoughtfully prepared into the feed on his page. Facebook meant so much to him. It elevated his life and gave him purpose. This was a platform for his politically incorrect jokes, his humorous comments, his caring and campaigning. He reconnected with schoolfriends, army mates, joined a community of fellow MND sufferers and befriended scores of people from around the world.

Before clicking the share tab, we read his final message together.

This says so much about Nigel. It illustrates his tremendous courage, his strength, determination and his irrepressible humour. He stresses his belief in self-determination, dignity and choice: sentiments championed by the 'Dignity in Dying' campaign, yet to impact on UK law. Never a man inclined to self-pity, or prepared to give in without a fight, he'd no intention of going quietly, either. Nigel's final words, these inspirational, uplifting words, will touch the hearts of many.

'That's going to set Facebook on fire,' says Becky.

'Not kidding,' says Ellie. 'Shame he won't get to see the comments.'

'No. He didn't want to spend his last few hours glued to Facebook,' I explain.

'Had to finish on a joke, didn't he?' remarks Craig.

I smile. 'Always.'

My hand hovers over the 'post' tab. 'Ready?'

'Go for it.'

I click the tab.

'It gives me great joy, today, to announce that I have found the one and only cure for MND, but it is with great sadness that it means I have had to go to Dignitas in Zurich to end my life.

'I would like to thank all my Facebook friends for their support and friendship since I joined in 2008, one year into this cruel illness. You have been a tremendous support to me throughout the ten years of this illness.

'It is such a shame that the laws of this country prevent me from doing this in my own home.

'My decision was arrived at because I wanted to take back control of my life and take the victory of killing me away from this disease. I wanted to die while I am happy and can still smile and not be controlled by this wicked disease any longer. I wanted to die with dignity instead of being tortured.

'Some people may think it's the easy way out but believe me it's not easy to leave your loving family and friends.

'I've been "dying" to post this! Ha ha ha ha ha!!

'Thank you and goodbye. XXX'

ACKNOWLEDGEMENTS

I have always dreamed of writing a book. I never expected the fulfilment of that dream to derive from such tragic circumstances.

When Nigel was ill with motor neurone disease, I started a blog. Partly as an escape from everyday existence and partly to search for the humour in it. As Nigel's condition worsened, I shared some of his experiences with our friends on Facebook. Thank you to those who took the time to read the posts and to those who made positive and encouraging comments – especially the readers who said, 'You should write a book.' This would later inspire me to develop those posts and do exactly that.

When I started writing this memoir, I was consumed by questions. What to include? What to leave out? How to structure it? How to make the scenes sing? I believe that, whatever the question, I'll find a book to point me in the direction of the answer. The first of many books I studied was Patti Miller's *Writing True Stories*. This practical resource proved invaluable in shaping my memoir. Then, the volumes of *The Writer's Lexicon,* by Kathy Steinemann, forced me to edit, edit and edit until I wanted to scream. But the grind resulted in a polished manuscript. These were just two of my helpers. My bookshelves now house an impressive collection of volumes which form my toolkit.

Nigel's was a story that simply had to be told. So, thanks must go to you Nigel, for refusing to leave my head. Your voice and laughter, anecdotes and jokes triggered a multitude of memories – most often when I was out walking Bodger – and propelled the book forward, page by page, chapter by chapter.

Writing a book is a lonely pastime, especially when, as a debut author, you haven't the confidence to tell people what you're doing. For a long time, the only person I confided in was my sister, Paula Stone. Paula, not only were you the keeper of my secret, but also the reader of every draft and redraft, giver of feedback and encouragement and staunch believer in my abilities. Without you, I am sure I would have given up. I am deeply grateful, Sis.

I am immensely grateful to our son, Craig Casson, and daughters Eleanor Collins and Rebecca Beattie, for trusting me to place them on the page and allowing me to share some of our most precious and private family moments. A special thanks to Rebecca, for taking the time to proofread the final draft and not demand a rewrite.

I am indebted to Nigel's brother, Les Casson, and sisters Tracey Casson and Melanie Armstrong, for unwittingly helping to shape the story as I wove our collective experiences into the narrative, and for your unquestioning support and patience once the book was written.

Thanks to all other family members who are represented in this book: Mum, Gloria Murgatroyd; daughter-in-law, Charlotte Casson; sons-in-law Danny Collins and Darryl Beattie; grandchildren, Ben Collins, Tom Collins, Jemma Casson and Amy Casson; brothers Nigel and Jez Murgatroyd; brothers-in-law Tom

Stone and Derek Armstrong; sister-in-law, Sally Casson and niece, Natalie Macrorie. This book would not be complete if you hadn't lived your part.

To friends Glyn Simpson; John Minford; Nigel Gamble (Gamby); Graham Forrest; Bruce Temple (RIP); Michele Lake and Rachel Bradshaw. I sincerely hope my recollection of those moments mirror yours.

Of course, without a publisher, there would be no book. My sincere thanks to Martin Hickman, owner of Canbury Press and Haythorp Books, for having enough faith in me to publish and present my book to the world. To Gabrielle Monteiro Machado, editing and marketing executive, and Jet Purdie for designing the cover. A special mention for my brother, Nigel Murgatroyd, for shooting the professional photograph which graces the cover.

My final and heartfelt thanks must go to you, dear reader. If you knew Nigel, I hope you recognised him in these pages, and smiled at your memories of him. If you didn't know him, I pray you were touched by the character and spirit of the man.

My greatest wish, for all of you, in reading Nigel's story, is for you to come to understand why he did what he did, to appreciate what drove him to make the choices he made, and to embrace and endorse his right to do so.

Perhaps one day, Nigel, your story will help to change the law in this country of ours.

JULIE CASSON

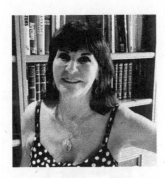

Julie Casson is a debut author. She is a mum, grandma and great-grandma and lives in Scarborough, North Yorkshire with her beloved miniature schnauzer Bodger.

Julie spent twenty-three years working in Further Education. Starting out as a teacher, her career evolved into management. She holds an MA in management from the University of York.

Her career ended unexpectedly in 2007, when her husband, Nigel, was diagnosed with motor neurone disease. Julie became Nigel's primary carer. Nigel's positivity, humour and pragmatism throughout his illness, and his determination to take control of his death, is the inspiration behind this memoir. In 2011, she started a blog, posting light-hearted commentary on every-day existence and specific accounts of Nigel's experience, which she later developed into this book. She completed a creative writing course with the University of York.

Julie is a supporter of the Motor Neurone Disease Association and member of Dignity in Dying.

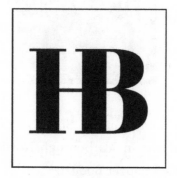

Publish with Us

We give writers the opportunity to see their work in print

We specialise in memoir, biography, autobiography and history,

but will consider other factual genres.

haythorp.co.uk

contact@haythorp.co.uk